Instructor's Manual/Test Bank/Transparency Masters

to accompany

McKenzie • Pinger

INTRODUCTION TO COMMUNITY HEALTH

Bonita L. McKenzie, M.Ed.
James F. McKenzie, Ph.D., M.P.H.
Robert R. Pinger, Ph.D.
Ball State University
Muncie, Indiana

Instructor's Manual/Test Bank/Transparency Masters to accompany McKenzie/Pinger,
INTRODUCTION TO COMMUNITY HEALTH

Copyright © 1995 by HarperCollins College Publishers

ISBN: 0-650-00798-0

95 96 97 98 99 9 8 7 6 5 4 3 2 1

Table of Contents

PREFACE

This combination instructor's manual and test bank was developed for professional educators who use INTRODUCTION TO COMMUNITY HEALTH. It was designed to assist individuals in preparing to teach the material contained in the textbook. Each chapter of this manual includes 1) a chapter synopsis, 2) a detailed chapter outline, 3) teaching ideas, 4) annotated references, and 5) annotated audiovisuals. Transparency masters are also provided to assist instructors in the presentation of the material. In addition, a test bank that includes a selection of multiple choice, true-false, matching, and short answer/essay questions and answers for each chapter is provided.

CHAPTER SYNOPSIS

The chapter synopsis provides a brief overview of the major concepts found in the chapter.

CHAPTER OUTLINE

A comprehensive outline is presented in the same order that the material is presented in the textbook. These pages may be used to provide you with a quick overview of the chapter content or they may be removed from this manual and used as actual lecture notes. Since each instructor has his or her own style of presenting material, space is provided within the outline for you to add your own ideas and reminders.

TEACHING IDEAS

There are countless ways that the content in each chapter can be presented. In the **Teaching Ideas** section of each chapter, we have offered some ideas we have found useful in presenting the material in our own classrooms.

ANNOTATED REFERENCES

This textbook is indeed an introduction to community health. Many of the topics that are covered in a chapter in the textbook have entire books written on them. As such, we identified a number of current useful books that can be 1) used to help you teach, 2) assigned as additional readings for the students, or 3) used as a source of references for student assignments.

ANNOTATED AUDIOVISUALS

There are a number of audiovisual materials on the market that could be very useful in presenting the material from the textbook to your students. In this section of each chapter, we have identified several items that can be used to supplement the material presented in the textbook. When available, we have provided an address for the producer of the audiovisuals.

TRANSPARENCY MASTERS

The final portion of the Instructor's Manual is a set of transparency masters of selected figures from the textbook.

TEST BANK

Following the Instructor's Manual you will find an extensive test bank with over 1,000 questions and answers. The test bank consists of multiple choice, true-false, matching, and short answer/essay questions for each chapter. Answer keys for each set of questions are provided. These questions are designed to be used alone or in addition to questions you create from your lectures and class activities. This test bank is also available from HarperCollins College Publishers to qualified adopters of INTRODUCTION TO COMMUNITY HEALTH on computer disks for both the Macintosh and DOS computers.

ACKNOWLEDGEMENTS

A project of this nature could not be completed without the assistance and understanding of a number of individuals. We would like to express our thanks to those individuals who took the time and effort to review this manuscript and provide feedback. In addition, we would like to acknowledge the assistance of the employees of HarperCollins College Publishers for the preparation of this project. Specifically, we would like to acknowledge the work of Bonnie Roesch, Director of Development and Executive Editor of Life Sciences, and Donna Campion, Supplements Editor of Life Sciences. Finally, we would like to express our deepest appreciation to Kathy Kennedy of Eta Sigma Gamma, Billie Kennedy and Ruth Ann Duncan of Ball State University, and Stephaney E. Pedler, a Ball State University student, for their help in preparing the manuscript.

Bonita L. McKenzie, M.Ed., James F. McKenzie, Ph.D., M.P.H., and Robert R. Pinger, Ph.D.

UNIT I

FOUNDATIONS OF COMMUNITY HEALTH

CHAPTER 1

Community Health--Yesterday, Today and Tomorrow

CHAPTER SYNOPSIS

In this introductory chapter, we introduce the concepts and principles of community health and explain the differences between community health and personal health and between community health and public health. Next we present a history of community health and public health. Finally we examine five serious health problems facing communities in the 1990s and offer an outlook for community health in the twenty-first century.

CHAPTER OUTLINE

I. Introduction

    A. Definitions

        1   Health is the blending of physical, emotional, social, intellectual, and spiritual resources as they assist in mastering the developmental tasks necessary to enjoy a satisfying and productive life.

        2. A community is a group of people with a shared location, shared environment and shared fate.

        3. Community health includes both private and public efforts of individuals, groups, and organizations to promote, protect and preserve the health of those in the community.

        4. Public health is the sum of all official (governmental) efforts to promote, protect and preserve the people's health.

    B. Roles of community health in society

        1. Personal health includes individual activities and decision making that affects the health of an individual or his or her family.

        2. Community health includes activities and planning aimed at protecting or improving the health of a community.

    C. Factors that affect the health of a community

        1. The physical factors that affect the community's health are geography, environment community size and industrial development.

2. The social and cultural factors that influence a community's health are beliefs, traditions, and prejudices, economies, politics, religion, social norms and socioeconomic status (SES).

3. The quality and effectiveness of community organization can affect the community's health.

4. Individual differences are often overlooked as an important influence on a community's health.

II. A Brief History of Community and Public Health

A. Evidence of community health practices can be traced to our earliest civilizations.

B. During the Middle Ages (500 to 1500 A.D.), little progress in public or community health was made and epidemics of communicable diseases were common.

C. The Period of Renaissance and Exploration (1500 to 1700 A.D.) brought a renewed interest in learning about causes and cures of diseases.

D. In the eighteenth century, a period characterized by industrial growth and poor sanitary conditions, epidemics of cholera, yellow fever and smallpox continued to ravage communities in both Europe and America.

E. The nineteenth century in America was characterized by westward expansion and a laissez-faire posture toward health issues by the government.

1. The beginning of the modern era of public health was marked by Lemual Shattuck's health report for the Commonwealth of Massachusetts in 1850.

2. The period of 1875-1900 has become known as the bacteriologic period of public health because during this period scientists discovered and described a great number of bacterial disease agents of communicable diseases.

F. The Twentieth Century

1. Health resources development period (1900-1960) was a period in which a number of medical schools, hospitals and nursing schools were built.

   a. The reform period (1900-1920) was characterized by social concerns which led Congress to pass legislation regulating the food and other industries.

   b. In the 1920s, prohibition resulted in a decline in alcohol related health problems.

   c. The Great Depression resulted in the passage of the Social Security Act of 1935, the first entry of the federal government into the welfare arena, and World War II resulted in a number of medical advances that would eventually be enjoyed by the civilian population.

   d. During the post war years, hospital construction resumed and attempts to plan national, state, and community health priorities failed.

2. The period of social engineering (1960-1975) saw the federal government take steps to improve access for the disadvantaged to health care.

        a.   Medicare

        b.   Medicaid

3.   The health promotion period (1975-1990) was a outgrowth of the discovery of the importance of lifestyle choices upon health.

4.   Community health in the 1990s faces at least five serious challenges.

        a.   <u>Health care delivery</u> and financing are a critical concern for the American people in the 1990s.

        b.   <u>Environmental problems</u> continued to be recognized as both economic and health issues.

        c.   <u>Lifestyle diseases</u> remain the leading killers of Americans.

        d.   As we enter the 1990s many scientists are recognizing that many <u>communicable diseases</u> such as AIDS, Lyme disease, tuberculosis and viral disease are still not conquered.

        e.   <u>Alcohol and other drug abuse</u> cost the country billions of dollars each year.

III. Outlook for Community Health in the Twenty-first Century

    A.   World Planning "Health for All by the Year 2000"

    B.   The United States Plan for Health in the Year 2000 -<u>Healthy People 2000.</u>

TEACHING IDEAS

Newspaper Clippings. Prior to presenting the content of this first chapter, scan your local newspaper looking for articles that are related to community health issues. Cut the articles out of the paper and have them made into overhead transparencies. At the appropriate time in the class show them to the students. Ask them if they feel if these are community health issues and ask them to defend their response based upon information presented in the text or class. Try to get the students to understand the difference between a community health issue and a personal health issue.

Writing Assignment. This activity could be conducted at the beginning or end of the lesson that covers the content in this chapter. Have the students identify what they think is the number one community health problem in their hometown, then have them defend their response. Have several students share their response, with the rest of the class and have the other students either agree or disagree with the rationale. If the activity is conducted at the beginning of the class it can be used at a springboard for the rest of the class time. If it is used at the end of the class, students can be asked to defend their response based on the information presented in text.

ANNOTATED REFERENCES

Cassedy, J.H. (1991). <u>Medicine in America: A short history.</u> Baltimore, MD: Johns Hopkins Press. The author divides the text into four time periods beginning with colonial times up to post 1940s. He discusses the medical profession, health related sciences, the government's role in health, health environment, and various health activities as they have related to the medical field.

Leviton, D. (Ed.). (1991). Horrendous death, health, and well-being. Bristol, PA: Hemisphere Publishing. The contents include the effects of horrendous death, defined as "man-made" death, on society. The three sections cover death by war, homicide, environmental destruction, poverty, accidents, and possible nuclear war.

Manning, W.G., et al. (1991). The costs of poor health habits. Cambridge, MA: Harvard University Press. This book is based on a RAND study and examines the costs of smoking, drinking, and lack of exercise. The authors include an explanation of the study's limitations and consider their own cost estimates conservative.

Rosen, G. (1993). A history of public health. Baltimore, MD: Johns Hopkins Press. Beginning chapters cover public health history before 1830. The focus, however, is on the recent past up to the beginning work of the World Health Organization and the United Nations.

Rosenberg, M.L., & Fenley, M.A. (Eds.). (1991). Violence in America: A public health approach. Cary, NC: Oxford University Press. Chapters in this book define the problem of violence, discuss specific forms of violence, and consider the epidemiology of violence, risk factors, causes, consequences, and intervention practices.

ANNOTATED AUDIOVISUALS

Churchill Media. Live or die. Los Angeles, CA: Author. Two fictional people who die at age 47 are profiled. The program describes how their lifestyles contributed to their early deaths. Also explained are habits that can lead to a healthy life. (32 minute videocassette)

Films for the Humanities and Sciences. Nature and nurture. Princeton, NJ: Author. [P.O. Box 2053, Princeton, NJ 08543-2053]. Issues concerning behavior tendencies at birth, chemical predispositions, and influences of environment are explored as they relate to the well-being of individuals. (52 minute videocassette)

Films for the Humanities and Sciences. Toward a livable city. Princeton, NJ: Author. [P.O. Box 2053, Princeton, NJ 08543-2053]. This video shows the development of Barcelona, Spain, from early history to recent growth. The program shows how government regulation of housing, transportation, air quality, fuel usage, and waste disposal has turned the city into a healthy, pleasant place to live. (24 minute videocassette)

Spectrum Films. For a change: breaking old habits and making new ones. Carlsbad, CA: Author. The program describes how to improve health through permanent behavior change. A systematic program shows ways to increase motivation, maintain records, set objectives, and sustain new behavior. (25 minute videocassette)

Spectrum Films. Health and lifestyle: positive approaches to well-being. Evanston, IL: Altschul Group Corporation. The relationship between health and lifelong habits is explored, emphasizing nutrition, weight control, exercise, and stress management. (28 minute videocassette)

CHAPTER 2

Organizations that Contribute to Community Health

CHAPTER SYNOPSIS

In Chapter 2, we discuss the need for the various health organizations that exist in our communities. We then describe each type of health agency and explain the differences in their purposes and responsibilities, their organizational structures and their funding.

CHAPTER OUTLINE

I. Introduction

    A. The size and complexity of today's communities hinder their ability to respond effectively to the health needs of their citizens unless they are organized for that purpose.

    B. There are several types of community health organizations: governmental, quasi-governmental, and nongovernmental.

II. Classification of Health Agencies

    A. Governmental (official) health agencies are funded by tax dollars and headed by government officials.

    B. Quasi-governmental health agencies receive funding from both public <u>and</u> private sources, and carry out functions expected of government agencies without government supervision.

    C. Nongovernmental (unofficial) health agencies are funded by private contributions and grants, and are not headed by government officials.

III. Governmental (Official) Health Agencies

    A. International health agencies

        1. The primary international health agency is the World Health Organization (WHO), founded in 1948.

        2. The WHO headquarters is located in Geneva, Switzerland.

        3. The primary operating body of WHO is the World Health Assembly, which comprises delegates from each of the member nations.

4. The purpose of WHO is to assist the peoples of member nations to attain the best level of health possible.

B. Federal health agencies

1. The lead health agency of the federal government is the <u>Department of Health & Human Services</u> (DHHS).

    a. Within DHHS, the Public Health Service (PHS) contributes most directly to community health. The PHS comprises the following agencies:

        1. The National Institutes of Health (NIH)

        2. The Food and Drug Administration (FDA)

        3. The Centers for Disease Control & Prevention (CDC)

        4. The Health Resources and Services Administration (HRSA)

        5. The Indiana Health Services (IHS)

        6. The Agency for Toxic Substances and Disease Registry (ATSDR)

        7. The Substance Abuse and Mental Health Services Administration (SAMHSA)

    b. The Health Care Financing Administration is responsible for administrating the Medicaid and Medicare programs.

    c. The Social Security Administration administers the Social Security Program.

    d. The Administration for Children and Families, the newest division of DHHS, coordinates the federal government's family programs and refugee assistance.

2. Other federal agencies also carry out health related activities.

    a. Department of Agriculture

    b. Department of Transportation

    c. Department of Labor

    d. Department of Interior

C. State health departments promote, protect and maintain the health and welfare of the citizens of the state.

D. Local health departments funded by local tax dollars provide health services to the people in their cities, counties and parishes. The organization and services provided vary greatly from location to location.

E. Comprehensive School Health Programs that include health education, a healthful school environment and health services can be considered official health agencies.

IV. Quasi-governmental Health Organizations

    A. The American Red Cross is the best known example of a quasi-governmental organization.

    B. There are similar agencies in many foreign countries.

V. Non-governmental (Unofficial) Health Agencies

    A. Voluntary health agencies are health organizations which were started by concerned citizens who saw a community health need not being met by any government agency.

       1. Voluntary health organizations often have national, state, and local offices.

       2. Among the best known are the American Cancer Society, the American Health Association, and Mothers Against Drunk Driving.

       3. Voluntary health agencies usually operate under a voluntary board of directors who hire a paid executive director who in turn directs a paid staff and a group of volunteers.

       4. The purposes of most voluntary health agencies are to raise money for research, educate the public and provide services to those in need.

    B. Professional health organizations/associations are funded by membership dues and serve to protect and promote the standards of the profession. Examples include the American Medical Association and the American Nursing Association.

    C. Philanthropic foundations provide money for projects and research to benefit society, much of it directed toward improving health. Examples are the Rockefeller Foundation, the Robert Wood Johnson Foundation and the Sloan-Kettering Foundation.

    D. Service organizations, such as the Shriners, Kiwanis, and Lion's clubs and religious groups often contribute significant health services to the community.

    E. Corporations affect the community's health through health and benefits packages, health and safety education programs and worksite fitness and recreation programs.

TEACHING IDEAS

Agency Health Fair. Assign each student or groups of students in your class to research a health agency. Then on a designated date have the students present their findings (complete with handouts and pamphlets from the agencies) to their classmates by setting up a "fair booth." The booth can be as elaborate as you wish, ranging from a table to a fully decorated exhibit. Have all the students visit the other booths in either a formal or informal mode.

Guest Speakers. Prior to the guest speakers coming to your classroom, have your students submit, in writing, a question that they would like the speakers to answer. This will help to prepare the students for the speakers and personalize the experience for them. After the class, have the students write a short one paragraph summary on what the speakers presented.

    1) Invite a "team" of employees in from a local health department. Try to get an administrator, a health educator, a public health nurse, and a sanitarian. Allow the speakers about half the time to talk about their jobs, responsibilities, and their organization and the other half of the time to answer questions.

2) Invite a panel of speakers to class that represent different voluntary health agencies. Ask each to take about 10 minutes to discuss research, education, and service in his/her agency, so that students can compare and contrast the different organizations.

ANNOTATED REFERENCES

Ashton, J. (Ed.). (1992). Healthy cities. Bristol, PA: Open University Press. Thirty-four writers describe the history and give an overview of the Healthy Cities Project developed by the WHO. The project's purpose was to promote effective practices for city health. It began with four cities, but has expanded to many others throughout the world.

Katz, A.H. (1993). Self-help in America: A social movement perspective. New York: Twayne Publishing. The author examines the reasons why self-help organizations have become so popular in today's society. He discusses the characteristics, dynamics and differences of and between 12-step and non-12-step organizations.

Richie, N.D., & Alperin, D.E. (1992). Innovation and change in the human services. Springfield, IL: Charles C. Thomas. This four part book summarizes the work of human service organizations (HSOs) in this century, explains trends and makes some predictions for new HSOs, offers a proposal for eliminating some problems in today's HSOs, and examines particular areas in HSOs that are expected to show substantial development.

White, K.L., et al. (Eds.). (1992). Health services research: An anthology (Scientific publication no. 534). Albany, NY: Pan American Health Organization. This anthology includes significant articles from the health services literature.

World Health Organization. (1990). Facts about WHO. Geneva, Switzerland: Author. This booklet includes an overview of the World Health Organization with information on its history, functions, achievements, challenges, goals, structure, and publications.

ANNOTATED AUDIOVISUALS

American Cancer Society. A mission statement. Atlanta, GA: Author. This program gives an overview of the work of the ACS, highlighting its work in the areas of service, education, and research. (7.5 minute videocassette) Note: Similar videocassettes are available from almost all voluntary health agencies. Check with the local offices.

ETV. A chance to live. Columbia, SC: Author. This program describes how the WHO and UNICEF worked to eliminate smallpox and immunize children against a number of communicable diseases. Also discussed is the importance of education concerning nutrition, birth control and AIDS in developing countries. (57 minute videocassette)

Rush/Winston Productions. American Red Cross emergency test. This video shows how to prepare for common emergency situations and presents the American Red Cross emergency test. (48 minute videocassette)

United Way of America. How United Way works. Alexandria, VA: Author. This program emphasizes that the United Way is a system for bringing people together to help address community needs. A profile of a homeless man who received assistance from a United Way agency and who is now living a meaningful life as a result, is shown. (10 minute videocassette)

World Health Organization. Health for all, all for health. Geneva, Switzerland: Author. This program traces the history of the World Health Organization (WHO) from its beginning in 1948 to the present. It shows how the WHO has worked to combat diseases in rich and poor countries within the past 40 years. (18 minute videocassette)

CHAPTER 3

Epidemiology: The Study of Disease, Injury and Death in the Community

CHAPTER SYNOPSIS

In Chapter 3, we define epidemiology and briefly review its history. We explain the importance of using rates to describe the occurrence of disease in populations and provide examples of different kinds of rates. We discuss several sources of standardized data and explain the three basic types of epidemiological studies.

CHAPTER OUTLINE

I. Introduction

    A. Epidemiology is the study of the distribution and determinants of disease and injury in human populations.

    B. Epidemics of communicable diseases have been common occurrences throughout history.

        1. It is possible to trace the history of epidemiology to ancient civilizations.

        2. The methods of epidemiology are important tools for public health professionals.

II. Rates

    A. Epidemiologists use rates to describe the occurrence and spread of diseases and health problems in populations.

    B. Three important kinds of rates are birth rates, death rates and morbidity rates.

    C. Incidence rates, prevalence rates and attack rates are important types of morbidity rates.

        1. An incidence rate is the number of <u>new</u> cases of a disease in a population at risk in a given period of time divided by the population.

        2. A prevalence rate is the number of <u>new</u> and <u>old</u> cases of a disease occurring at a given point of time divided by the population.

        3. An attack rate is a special incidence rate calculated for a particular population for a single disease outbreak and expressed as a percent.

D. Crude and specific rates

   1. For crude rates the entire population is the denominator.

   2. Specific rates measure the rates of specific diseases, or diseases in specific populations.

III. Reporting of Births, Deaths and Disease

   A. All births and deaths, as well as all cases of certain notifiable diseases occurring in the United States, must be reported to health authorities.

   B. Local, state and federal governments maintain vital and disease records which can be used by epidemiologists and other health professionals to track and study disease.

IV. Sources of Standardized Data

   A. The U.S. Census, conducted every ten years, is an enumeration of the population living in the United States and provides useful demographic information to health workers.

   B. The Statistical Abstract of the United States is a summary of useful statistics on the social, political and economic organization of the United States.

   C. Vital Statistics are statistical summaries of records of major life events.

   D. Morbidity and Mortality Weekly Report lists cases of notifiable diseases in the United States.

V. Epidemilogical Studies

   A. Descriptive studies describe the extent of a disease outbreak with regard to person, place and time.

   B. Analytical studies test hypotheses about relationships between health problems and possible risk factors.

   1. Retrospective studies (case control studies) compare people with disease (cases) to healthy people of similar age, sex and background (controls), with respect to prior exposure to possible risk factors.

   2. Prospective studies (cohort studies) are studies in which subjects that belong to a large group of similar experience (a cohort) are classified by exposure to certain risk factors and observed into the future to determine disease outcomes.

   C. Experimental studies seek to identify the cause of disease or effectiveness of a treatment by controlling all or most of the variables surrounding the experimental subjects. Experimental studies typically adhere to the following principles: control groups, randomization and blindness.

   1. Control groups receive a placebo treatment.

   2. Experimental subjects are assigned to control and treatment groups randomly.

3. In a properly designed experiment, subjects and researchers remain uninformed (blind) as to the identity of treatment and control groups until after data are recorded.

TEACHING IDEAS

Newspaper Obituaries. Have your students read the obituaries from a newspaper for a period of two weeks. As they read the obituaries, have them record the age, sex, and cause of death for each person noted. Then have your students multiple the data by 26 to give them an equivalent of one years worth of data. Let the students calculate crude mortality rates, and cause and age specific mortality rates.

Guest Speaker. Invite an epidemiologist in from the local health department or hospital. Ask him/her to explain his/her work, the importance of the work, what a typical day of work is like, and present some of the more interesting cases on which he/she has worked. Then open the session up to questions.

ANNOTATED REFERENCES

Duncan, D.F. (1988). Epidemiology: Basis for disease prevention and health promotion. New York: Macmillan Publishing Co. This is a good source for students, providing basic information on epidemiology. The text includes background information on epidemiology, statistical methods, epidemiologic distributions, and epidemiologic research.

Elliot, P. et al. (Eds.). (1992). Geographical and environmental epidemiology: Methods for small-area studies. New York: Oxford University Press. International experts discuss issues and techniques of environmental and geographical epidemiology. The book's five sections include: an introduction to geographical and small area studies, data requirements, statistical methods, a historical overview, and case histories of small-area and geographical studies.

Harper, A.C., & Lambert, L. (1994). The health of populations: An introduction. New York: Springer Publishing Co. This text gives an easy to understand overview of epidemiology. The authors explain the determinants of the health of a community and give a history of the development of population health.

Mausner, J.S., & Kramer, S. (1985). Mausner & Bahn Epidemiology -An introductory text. (6th ed.). Philadelphia, PA: W.B. Saunders. This textbook was designed to provide a background in epidemiology for students enrolled in an introductory course in epidemiology, community medicine, health administration, or public health. Though a bit dated, the book includes the basics of epidemiology using certain diseases and problems as illustrations.

Timmreck. (1994). An introduction to epidemiology. Boston, MA: Jones and Bartlett Publishers. This is a good reference for health professionals, giving an overview and comprehensive look at epidemiology.

ANNOTATED AUDIOVISUALS

American Academy of Pediatrics. A gift, an obligation. Evanston, IL: Author. [1801 Hinman Ave., Evanston, IL, 60204]. This is a program to inform people of the dangers of childhood diseases and to encourage parents to make sure that their children are fully immunized. (30 minute 16 mm film) [Note: This film could also be used with Chapters 6 or 8]

BBC-TV Production. <u>Riddle of the joints</u>. Northbrook, IL: Coronet Film and Video. The program looks at the history as well as recent research on rheumatoid arthritis. The breakdown of the immune system is examined as a possible cause. The human parvavirus and Lyme disease are also studied as possible causes of arthritis. (58 minute videocassette)

Filmakers Library. <u>The White Plague: Tuberculosis</u>. NY: Author. [124 East 40th St., New York, NY 10016]. This production discusses the increase of TB in the United States, and suggests that the disease is reaching plague proportions in some major cities. It offers reasons and conditions for this outbreak and also studies the problem of drug resistant TB. (45 minute videocassette)

PBS Video. <u>Plagues</u>. Alexandria, VA: Author. The program is presented by Baruch S. Blumberg, Nobel laureate. He examines modern plagues; how they have spread and changed lives. Also discussed are the outbreak of cholera in London in the nineteenth century, and the epidemics of influenza, legionnaires' disease, myxomatosis, and malaria. (59 minute videocassette)

CHAPTER 4

Epidemiology: Prevention and Control of Diseases and Health Conditions

CHAPTER SYNOPSIS

In this chapter we present a classification of diseases and other health problems and provide examples of diseases in each classification. Models for communicable disease transmission are presented and explained as is a model for multicausation disease. We discuss ways communities can prioritize health problems and then define terms used in disease prevention and control. Lastly, we discuss primary, secondary, and tertiary prevention as it applies to both communicable and noncommunicable diseases.

CHAPTER OUTLINE

I.   Introduction

    A.   Epidemiologic fundamentals were presented in Chapter Three.

    B.   Chapter Four provides principles of prevention and control of diseases.

II. Classification of Diseases and Health Problems

    A.   Communicable vs. noncommunicable diseases

        1.   Communicable diseases are caused by pathogenic agents which can be transmitted from an infected host to a noninfected, susceptible one.

        2.   Noncommunicable diseases cannot be transmitted from a diseased host to a susceptible one.

    B.   Acute vs. chronic diseases and illnesses

        1.   With acute diseases, the peak severity of symptoms occurs within three months of the onset of the illness.

        2.   Chronic diseases last longer than three months, sometimes for the remainder of one's life.

III. Communicable Diseases

    A.   The communicable disease model includes the three basic elements involved: the communicable disease agent, host and environment.

B. The <u>chain of infection</u> is a model that conceptualizes the transmission of a communicable disease from its source to a new susceptible host.

C. Modes of transmission include <u>direct</u> and <u>indirect transmission</u>.

    1. Direct transmission includes touching, sneezing and sexual contact.

    2. Indirect transmission can be air-borne, water-borne, vehicle-borne or vector-borne.

IV. Noncommunicable Diseases

A. Noncommunicable disease can best be visualized by the multi-causation disease model.

B. Diseases of the heart and blood vessels are the leading cause of death in America.

    1. coronary heart disease

    2. cerebrovascular accidents

C. Malignant neoplasms kill more than one-half million people annually in the U.S.

D. Other noncommunicable disease problems

    1. chronic obstructive pulmonary disease

    2. diabetes mellitus

    3. chronic liver disease and cirrhosis

    4. others

V. Prioritizing Prevention and Control Efforts

A. Leading causes of death is perhaps the most common way people prioritize health problems.

B. Years of Potential Life Lost (YPLL) is a measurement that emphasizes the importance of those diseases that kill at an early age.

C. Economic cost to society of various health problems is yet another way to prioritize health problems.

VI. Prevention, Intervention, Control, and Eradication of Diseases

A. <u>Prevention</u> is the taking of action to prevent or forestall the onset of illness or injury before pathogenesis.

B. <u>Intervention</u> is the taking of action to control a disease in progress.

C. Control means that containment of a disease and can include both prevention and intervention measures.

D. <u>Eradication</u> is the uprooting or total elimination of a disease from the human population.

VII. Levels of Prevention

    A. Primary prevention is the forestalling of the onset of illness or injury during the pre-pathogenesis period (before the disease process begins).

    B. Secondary prevention is the early diagnosis and prompt treatment of diseases before the disease becomes advanced and disability becomes severe.

    C. Tertiary prevention is to retrain, reeducate and rehabilitate the patient who has already incurred disability.

    D. Prevention of Communicable Diseases

        1. primary prevention of communicable diseases

        2. secondary prevention of communicable diseases

        3. tertiary prevention of communicable diseases

        4. application of preventive measures for the control of a communicable disease: HIV/AIDS

            a. chain of infection

            b. universal precautions

    E. Prevention of Noncommunicable Diseases

        1. primary prevention of noncommunicable diseases

        2. secondary prevention of noncommunicable diseases

        3. tertiary prevention of noncommunicable diseases

        4. application of preventive measures for the control of a noncommunicable disease: CHD

            a. the community's role

            b. the individual's role

TEACHING IDEAS

Oral Presentation. Have the students select a disease to research for an oral presentation. Instruct the students to find information so they can present the following in a 15 minute presentation to the class: overview of the disease (who it affects, seriousness of the disease, cost to society, cause of the disease), classification of the disease, means of spreading (use chain of infection if appropriate), means of prevention, and a prediction for eradicating the disease.

Application of Disease Prevention. After you have presented the information contained in this chapter, select a couple of communicable and noncommunicable diseases and with the help of your students develop a prevention strategy for each. Consider all three levels of prevention and discuss both the individual's and community's role.

ANNOTATED REFERENCES

Beneson, A.S. (Ed.). (1990). Control of communicable diseases in man. Washington D.C.: APHA. This manual covers information on over 200 communicable diseases. Information on each disease includes: identification, infectious agent, where and how it is contracted, incubation, susceptibility, resistance, control, and prevention.

Crowley, L.V. (1992). Introduction to human disease. Boston, MA: Jones and Bartlett Publishers. This text includes information on the structural and functional changes brought on by disease, and explains the principles of treatment. Two sections describe diseases and their effects on the body as a whole and on individual organ systems.

Morse, S.S. (Ed.). (1993). Emerging viruses. New York: Oxford University Press. This text discusses the emergence and evolution of viruses by looking at some representative viruses. Authors provide information on: history of viral emergence, the relationship between virus and host, detection and tracking of emerging viruses.

National Safety Council. (1993). Bloodborne pathogens. Boston: Jones and Bartlett Publishers. This text is a teaching program alerting students in health fields of the risk of exposure to bloodborne pathogens, such as HIV and hepatitis B virus. At the end of each chapter are learning activities to reinforce content and test knowledge.

U.S. Department of Health and Human Services & Public Health Service. (1990). Healthy people 2000. Washington, D.C.: U.S. Government Printing Office. This government publication is a comprehensive source that studies our nation's health at the present time and discusses objectives for a healthier future population. The text studies the concepts of personal responsibility for health, the creation of a "culture of character," especially in the poorer segments of society, health promotion, and disease prevention.

ANNOTATED AUDIOVISUALS

Coastal Health Care. Tuberculosis: back from the past. Virginia Beach: VA: Author. The appearance of tuberculosis is examined as well as the resistance of new strains of the disease to many drugs. Also discussed are transmission of the disease, environmental and work practice controls, and personal protection. (18 minute videocassette)

Colossal Entertainment, Inc. Cancer: we can beat it! Atlanta, GA: Author. This video studies the causes, symptoms, risk factors, and prevention practices for a variety of types of cancer. (38 minute videocassette)

Films for the Humanities & Sciences. Intimate epidemic. Princeton, NJ: Author. [P.O. Box 2053, Princeton, NJ 08543-2053]. This videocassette examines the epidemic of sexually transmitted diseases; gonorrhea, syphilis, herpes, chlamydia, genital warts, and HIV/AIDS. Epidemiologists offer information concerning advances in detecting, treating, and preventing these diseases. (24 minute videocassette)

Films for the Humanities & Sciences. Sexually transmitted diseases. Princeton, NJ: Author. [P.O. Box 2053, Princeton, NJ 08543-2053].This program emphasizes prevention and early detection of STDs: chlamydia, herpes, veneral warts, and AIDS. The video also looks at the consequences of these diseases, such as: infertility, tubal pregnancy and infections in infants. (19 minute videocassette)

Time-Life Video. Death of a disease. New York: Author. This program explains how smallpox has been eliminated throughout the world through the efforts of the WHO. The campaign began in 1967 through widespread vaccination. (58 minute videocassette)

CHAPTER 5

Community Organization and Health Promotion Planning: Two Important Tools of Community Health

CHAPTER SYNOPSIS

In Chapters 3 and 4, we described epidemiological methods, which are essential tools for the community health professional. In this chapter, we describe two additional skills useful to the community health values: how to organize a community and how to plan a community health program.

CHAPTER OUTLINE

I. Introduction

    A. Little in the way of community health can be achieved unless the community health professional understands the dynamics of community organization.

    B. Among the most important skills is the ability to plan a community health promotion/disease prevention program.

II. Community Organization

    A. Community organization and community development are similar terms that have different meanings.

        1. Community organization is "intervention whereby individuals, groups, and organizations engage in planned action to influence social problems. It is concerned with the enrichment, development, and/or change of social institutions."

        2. Community development is "a mass process designed to create conditions of economic and social progress for a whole community with its active participation and the fullest possible reliance on the community's initiative."

    B. There are seven assumptions for community organization.

        1. Communities of people can develop capacity to deal with their own problems.

        2. People want to change and can change.

        3. People should participate in making, adjusting, or controlling the major changes taking place in their communities.

4. Changes in community living that are self-imposed or self-developed have a meaning and permanence that imposed changes do not have.

5. A 'holistic approach' can deal successfully with problems with which a 'fragmented approach' cannot cope.

6. Democracy requires cooperative participation and action in the affairs of the community, and people must learn the skills which make this possible.

7. Frequently, communities of people need help in organizing to deal with their needs, just as many individuals require help in coping with their individual problems.

C. Three approaches to community organization have proven successful.

1. Locality development is a broad self-help method in which local citizens develop new skills and become more self-sufficient.

2. Social planning utilizes skilled volunteers in the community in a technical process of problem solving.

3. Social action is a technique that involves the redistribution of power and resources to disadvantaged segments of the population.

III. Organizing a Community: A Process

A. Recognizing a community health problem.

B. Gaining entry into the community.

C. Organizing the people.

D. Identifying the specific problem through a needs assessment.

E. Determining priorities and setting goals.

F. Arriving at a solution and selecting intervention activities.

G. The Final Steps in the Process.

1. Implementation is the execution of the intervention activities.

2. Evaluation of results reveals the degree of success.

3. Maintaining the intervention long enough to ensure success.

4. Looping back to an earlier stage of the plan, if necessary

IV. Health Promotion and Disease Prevention Programming

A. Health promotion/disease prevention program planning can trace its roots to the 1979 Surgeon General's Report on Health, Promotion and Disease Prevention.

B. Basic understanding of program planning involves understanding that:

1. <u>Health education</u> is the "the continuum of learning which enables people, as individuals and as members of social structures, to voluntarily make decisions, modify behaviors, and change social conditions in ways that are health enhancing."

2. <u>Health promotion/disease prevention</u> is "the aggregate of all purposeful activities designed to improve personal and public health through a combination of strategies, including the competent implementation of behavioral change strategies, health education, health protection measures, risk factor detection, health enhancement and health maintenance."

3. <u>Program planning</u> is a process in which an intervention is planned to help meet the needs of a specific group of people.

4. <u>Community organization</u> is "intervention whereby individuals, groups, and organizations engage in planned action to influence social problems. It is concerned with the enrichment, development, and/or change of social institutions."

V. Creating a Health Promotion/Disease Prevention Program

A. <u>Assessing the needs</u> of the target population is the first task in creating a health promotion/disease prevention program.

1. Step 1 is determining the present state of health of the target population.

2. Step 2 is identifying existing programs.

3. Step 3 is comparing health deficits with existing programs.

4. Step 4 is dealing with the problems.

5. Step 5 is validating the need.

B. <u>Setting goals and objectives</u> is laying the foundation for the program.

C. <u>Developing an intervention</u> is designing the activities that will help the target population meet their objectives

D. <u>Implementing the intervention</u> is the actual putting into practice of the activities that made up the intervention.

E. <u>Evaluating the results</u> is comparing the program's outcome with some standard of acceptability. The process involves five steps.

1. Planning the evaluation

2. Collecting the data

3. Analyzing the data

4. Reporting results

5. Applying the results

TEACHING IDEAS

Simulation. Create a simulation of a community organization effort in a community to help the students understand the difficulty of bringing a group of people together. Select an issue like "no smoking in public places." Then assign different roles to the members of the class such as health educator, tobacco farmer, avid smoker, avid non-smoker, a retailer who sells tobacco, a restaurant owner, and any others you think would be interesting. Have each student make a five minute presentation on his/her point of view on the issue. Then as a class discuss the steps of the community organization process considering the presentation of the students.

Guest Speaker. Invite a person to class that has been responsible for developing a health promotion program. Ask the speaker to address each of the steps in the planning process as it related to the program he/she planned.

ANNOTATED REFERENCES

Butler, J.T. (1994). Principles of health education and health promotion. Englewood, CO: Morton Publishing Company. This textbook, which is focused at pre-service health educators and health promoters, was written to provide a clear, succinct guide to the fields of health education and health promotion. It presents information on the role of the health educator, the settings for health education, theories of health behavior, and the components of program planning, implementation, and evaluation.

Chenoweth, D.H. (1991). Planning health promotion at the worksite. (2nd edition). Champaign, IL: Brown & Benchmark. Part I of this text focuses on the planning of worksite health promotion including a rationale, the designing of the program planning process, implementation, and evaluation. Part II discusses the professional preparation for worksite health promotion. Appendices include information such as: the Kansas City Model Plan, marketing basics, key resources, sample outlines, consent form, sample program advertisements.

Dignan, M.B., & Carr, P.A. (1987). Program planning for health education and health promotion. Philadelphia, PA: Lea & Febiger. In six chapters, this book presents a comprehensive model for planning and evaluating community health programs. The specific components of the model include community analysis, program focus, program development, program implementation, and program evaluation.

Gilmore, G., Campbell, M.D., & Becker, B.L. (1989). Needs assessment strategies for health education and health promotion. Madison, WI: Brown & Benchmark. This text begins with an overview of needs assessment strategies. The authors then discuss assessments with individuals, assessments with groups, self-directed assessments, case studies, and a computer simulation.

Green, L.W., & Kreuter, M.W. (1991). Health promotion planning: An educational and environmental approach. Mountain View, CA: Mayfield Publishing. This textbook, written by two of the most respected health educators in the United States, presents the best known and most-widely distributed health promotion planning model; PRECEDE/PROCEED. The model is explained in great detail with individual chapters dedicated to each of the phases of the model. In addition, the text provides a number of examples of the model's application.

McKenzie, J.F., & Jurs, J.L. (1993). Planning, implementing, and evaluating health promotion programs: A primer. New York: Macmillan Publishing Company. This textbook is designed to provide the student with the knowledge to develop the skills necessary to plan, carry out, and evaluate health promotion programs regardless of the setting. It is unique among other program-planning health textbooks in that it provides readers with both the theoretical and practical information. This text also includes a chapter on community organization.

Opatz, J.P. (Ed.). (1994). Economic impact of worksite health promotion. Champaign, IL: Human Kinetics Publishers. The three parts of this text include: theory concerning worksite health promotion, the definition of worksite health promotion, a review and evaluation of current studies, a nine step model for planning a program evaluation, and specific case studies. This book is a publication of the Association for Worksite Health Promotion.

Sarvela, P.D., & McDermott, R.J. (1993). Health education evaluation and measurement: A practitioner's perspective. Madison, WI: WCB Brown & Benchmark Publishers. This is a "user-friendly" textbook that presents the basic information concerning evaluation and measurement. Readers are provided with the opportunity to apply the material by responding to the case studies, questions and activities at the end of each chapter.

ANNOTATED AUDIOVISUALS

Association for the Advancement of Health Education. Health education work! Reston, VA: Author. [1900 Association Drive, Reston, VA 22091]. This videocassette program answers the question "Does health education work"? According to the video the answer is YES! Examples of successful health education programs in four different settings (schools, community, clinical, and worksites) are presented. Also the five key components of successful programs are noted. They include: (1) careful planning, (2) focus on modifiable risk factors, (3) use of multiple intervention strategies, (4) involving the target population in the planning, and (5) qualified personnel to conduct the programs. (15 minute videocassette) [Note: This videocassette could also be used with Chapter 6]

Films for the Humanities & Sciences. AIDS, the family and the community. Princeton, NJ: Author. [P.O. Box 2053, Princeton, NJ 08543-2053]. This program gives an overview of AIDS, and focuses on the importance of community support for patients and their families, whether the setting is urban or rural. (26 minute videocassette)

Health Promotion Resource Center at Stanford University. Community health promotion: a program in action. Palo Alto, CA: Author. The videocassette looks at the Stanford Heart Disease Prevention Program and how community health promotion principles were applied to this program. (48 minute videocassette)

IOX Videotape Division. Fundamentals of program evaluation for health educators. Culver City, CA: Author. [14111 West Jefferson Blvd., Culver City, CA, 90230]. This videocassette features Drs. Donald C. Iverson and W. James Popham as they discuss four features of program evaluation: (1) the function of program evaluation, (2) data gathering designs, (3) appropriate measuring instruments, and (4) effective use of sampling. After the presentation of each section a short quiz is presented to check learning. (45 minute videocassette)

Learning Multi-Systems, Inc. Drug free zones...Taking action. Madison, WI: Author. [320 Holtzman Rd., Madison, WI 53713]. This program offers methods and solutions communities can use to fight drug and alcohol related problems in schools, neighborhoods, parks, and housing developments. (27 minute videocassette)

CHAPTER 6

The School Health Program: A Component of Community Health

CHAPTER SYNOPSIS

The school health program is an important component of community health because every citizen must pass through this institution. In this chapter, we define school health and the roles of those involved in the delivery of school health programs. We also discuss the development and implementation of school health policy and describe the major components of an ideal school health program. Lastly, we examine the major issues facing school health today.

CHAPTER OUTLINE

I. Introduction

    A. A <u>comprehensive school health program</u> is an organized set of policies, procedures and activities designed to protect and promote the health and well-being of students and staff. The three components are:

        1. School health services

        2. Healthful school environment

        3. Health education

    B. The <u>school health team</u> should include representation from administrators, food service workers, counseling, personnel, maintenance workers, medical personnel, social workers, parents, students and teachers.

    C. The <u>school nurse</u> is in position to provide leadership in the school health program and usually has the following responsibilities.

        1. Maintain and review birth records

        2. Dispense medications

        3. Train others

        4. Conduct health follow-ups

        5. Help develop school health policies

6. Identify students with medical problems

7. Identify community resources for school health

D. The teacher's role is to understand and facilitate the school health program, to provide health instruction that is meaningful and to identify behavioral conditions that suggest health problems in students.

II. **Why School Health?**

A. Children with nutritional or other health problems are less able to learn.

B. Healthy People 2000 objectives reflect the importance of school health programs.

III. **Foundations of the School Health Program**

A. Well organized, genuinely interested school health team.

B. Supportive administration

C. Qualified personnel

IV. **School Health Policies**

A. School health policies are written statements used to guide those who work with the program.

B. The school health policy is developed by the school health team and overall aspects of the school health program.

C. Policy implementation requires the following steps:

1. Distribution

2. Placement in school handbooks

3. Presentation at a meeting

V. **Major Components of a Comprehensive School Health Program**

A. Administration and organization of the policy includes coordination of the program by a knowledgeable individual such as the school nurse.

B. School Health Services comprise health appraisals, emergency services, prevention and control of communicable diseases, provision for handicapped students, health advising and remediation of detected health problems.

C. The healthful school environment facet of the comprehensive school health programs provides for a safe and healthful learning environment.

1. The physical environment includes location and age of buildings, lighting, heating, acoustics, water supply, sanitation and food service provided to the school community.

2. The social/emotional environment includes less tangible characteristics of the school such as friendliness, politeness and respectful behavior of teachers and students.

D. <u>Health instruction</u> is the development, delivery, and evaluation of a planned curriculum.

   1. Approaches to designing an instructional curriculum include:

      a. <u>Direct instruction</u>, in which health is taught as a separate discipline

      b. <u>Correlated instruction</u>, in which health is taught as a part of other disciplines, i.e. science, home economics or physical education.

      c. <u>Integrated instruction</u>, in which health is the vehicle through which other disciplines are taught.

   2. Curriculum development occurs at the local, state or national levels.

   3. There are several curriculum models that have received national recognition.

      a. <u>Growing Healthy</u>

      b. <u>Have a Healthy Heart</u>

      c. <u>Teenage Health Teaching Modules</u>

      d. <u>School Health Education Study</u>

VI. Issues and Concerns Facing the School Health Program

A. Comprehensive school health programs are not in place in all schools although the need remains strong.

B. Controversy over school health curricula are based on differing values and religious teachings and over the proper implementing of the curriculum.

C. School-based clinics or school-linked clinics provide students with comprehensive health care services at or adjacent to schools.

TEACHING IDEAS

Class Debate. After you have presented the material contained in this chapter, divide the class in half to debate the issue of whether or not health education should be taught in each grade K-12. Have each side research the issue, but give them some ideas on which to build their case. Included may be things like: other subjects (i.e., math, English, etc.) are taught K-12, we have gotten along okay to date without comprehensive school health so why now, there is no time in the school day for another class, health issues should be taught at home not in school, etc.

Guest Panel. Invite to your class the members of a school health team from a local school district. Have each panel member provide an overview of his/her responsibilities as a member of the team. Then have the panel share with the class the issues they have faced. If panel members do not address controversial issues, have a talk about the implementation of sex education curriculum or starting a school based clinic.

ANNOTATED REFERENCES

Cornacchia, H.J., Olsen, L.K., & Nickerson, C.J. (1988). Health in elementary schools. (7th ed.). St. Louis, MO: Times Mirror/Mosby College Publishing. This book has been designed to be a practical guide for prospective and in-service elementary teachers and for health service personnel and school administrators. It presents an overview of the school health program, outlines the teacher's role in school health, and provides in depth coverage of healthful school living, health services, health education, methods of teaching health, and evaluation of the school health program.

Creswell, Jr., W.H., & Newman, I.M. (1993). School health practice. (10th ed.). St. Louis: Mosby - Year Book, Inc. This book was written for elementary and secondary level school teachers, specialists in health education, school social workers, school psychologists, school health service personnel, and school administrators. Since this text was published after Healthy People 2000, it includes many references to the national health promotion and disease prevention objectives. The major sections of the book include: organization of the school health program, the school-age child, school health services, health instruction, healthful school living, and appraisals in school health practice.

Meeks, L.B., & Heit, P. (1992). Comprehensive school health education: Totally awesome strategies for teaching health. Blacklick, OH: Meeks Heit Publishing Company. This book was developed to include everything that pre-service and in-service teachers need to implement a comprehensive school health program. It references the Healthy People 2000 objectives. Key components of the book include sections on a framework for comprehensive school health education, background information and totally awesome strategies for teaching health, totally awesome teaching masters and student masters, and resources that enhance the teaching of health.

Pollock, M.B., & Middleton, K. (1994). School health instruction: The elementary and middle school years. (3rd ed.). St. Louis: Mosby - Year Book, Inc. The third edition of this book remains one designed to help prospective elementary and middle school teachers teach children what they want and need to know about their health. The overall intent of the book is to provide the concepts and basic skills needed to understand, plan, and carry out a curriculum that reflects the very best of what is known about effective health teaching today. It also presents information on the role of health services and provisions in protecting the safety and sanitation of the school's environment.

Redican, K.J., Olsen, L.K., & Baffi, C.R. (1986). Organization of school health programs. New York: Macmillan Publishing Co. Although this book is a bit dated, it still contains information that can be very useful for those wanting greater depth in organizing a school health program. The text is divided into four major sections including foundations, school health environment, school health services, and health instruction.

ANNOTATED AUDIOVISUALS

American Academy of Pediatrics. A gift, an obligation. Evanston, IL: Author. [1801 Hinman Ave., Evanston, IL, 60204]. This is a program to inform people of the dangers of childhood diseases and to encourage parents to make sure that their are fully immunized. (30 minute 16 mm film) [Note: This film could also be used with Chapters 3 or 8]

Association for the Advancement of Health Education. Health education work! Reston, VA: Author. [1900 Association Drive, Reston, VA 22091]. This videocassette program answers the question "Does health education work"? According to the video, the answer is YES! Examples of successful health education programs in four different settings (schools, community, clinical, and worksites) are presented. Also the five key components of successful programs are noted. They include: (1) careful planning, (2) focus on modifiable risk factors, (3) use of multiple intervention strategies, (4) involving the target population in the planning, and (5) qualified personnel to conduct the programs. (15 minute videocassette) [Note: This videocassette could also be used with Chapter 5]

Metropolitan Life Foundation. Healthy me. New York, NY: Author. [Health and Safety Education Division, One Madison Ave., NY, NY, 10010]. This videocassette emphasizes the importance of comprehensive school health by showing a number of schools that offer such. Healthy Me is a program of the Metropolitan Life Foundation to support school health. The foundation presents case awards to schools that can serve as models and to community groups who support comprehensive school health. (18 minute videocassette)

Metropolitan Life Foundation. You can see tomorrow. New York, NY: Author. [Health and Safety Education Division, One Madison Ave., NY, NY, 10010]. This program is a documentary film intended to help teachers and parents to be more aware of their children's health, and to encourage them to take appropriate action when required. The film not only focuses on the prevention and recognition of problems such as vision, hearing, nutrition, infectious diseases and allergies, but also touches on emotional and behavioral issues. (30 minute 16 mm film). [Note: This film could also be used with Chapter 8]

The National Center for Health Education. Growing healthy. Studio City, CA: Film Fair Communications. [10900 Ventura Blvd., Studio City, CA]. This videocassette provides an overview of the comprehensive K-7 health education curriculum Growing Healthy. It presents examples of schools where the curriculum has been implemented. It also explains how teachers are trained in the curriculum and how the curriculum is funded. (23 minute videocassette)

UNIT II

THE NATION'S HEALTH

CHAPTER 7

A Health Profile of the American People

CHAPTER SYNOPSIS

The chapter provides an overview of the health status of Americans using a broadly constructed age-group classification: infants and children, adolescents and young adults, adults, and seniors. This survey is preceded by a review and explanation of various measures of health status including mortality rates, life expectancy, years of potential life lost and other measures of health.

CHAPTER OUTLINE

I.   Introduction

II. Health Status and Its Measurement

    A.   Mortality statistics are among the most accurate statistics available.

        1.   They provide helpful information about leading causes of death.

        2.   They can be used to rank important health problems.

    B.   Life expectancy data are useful for comparing the healthiness of the community and of different sub-populations within the community.

    C.   Years of potential life lost (YPLL) is a health statistic that preferentially emphasizes deaths of the young more heavily than deaths of the elderly.

    D.   National health interview survey data are self-reported data about the respondents' health status.

    E.   National health and nutrition examination survey is conducted by the National Center for Health Statistics to assess the health and nutritional status of Americans.

    F.   <u>Disability Adjusted Life Years</u> (DALYs) is a measure that combines loss from premature mortality and loss of healthy life resulting from disability.

III. Creating a Health Profile of Americans Requires Examining the Population by Age Group

IV. The Health Profile of Infants and Children

    A.   Infant mortality is an important measure of the health of a community and of sub-populations within that community.

B. Childhood health is a measure of parenting skills as well as quality of communities' health services.

C. The threat of deaths from infectious diseases has declined during the past 40 years.

V. The Health Profile of Adolescents and Young Adults

A. Overall mortality rates for the 15-24 year age group have declined in the past 40 years by 19%.

1. Deaths from unintentional and intentional injuries are the leading causes of death.

2. Homicide and suicide rates have increased in recent years.

B. Morbidity rises from communicable diseases such as measles, gonorrhea, AIDS and syphilis.

C. Health behavior and lifestyle choices are made during this age--decision about diet, exercise, alcohol, tobacco and other drug use.

1. Experimentation with alcohol and other drugs peaks during these years.

2. Use of tobacco products represents one of the most serious health problems for this group.

3. Physical fighting and weapon carrying are a growing concern.

4. Sexual activity, resulting in unintended pregnancies and disease transmission, lowers the health status of this age group.

VI. The Health Profile of Adults

A. Mortality rates for adults have declined significantly over the past 40 years.

1. Noncommunicable diseases remain the leading causes of death.

   a. Cancer

      1. Lung cancer

      2. Colorectal cancer

      3. Breast cancer

   b. Cardiovascular diseases

   c. Other leading causes of death

      1. Injuries

      2. Diseases of the liver

      3. Respiratory diseases

      4. HIV/AIDS

　　　　　　5.　Diabetes

　　　2.　Health behavior and lifestyle choices involve reducing risks for certain chronic diseases.

　　　　　　a.　Smoking cessation

　　　　　　b.　Dietary choices

　　　　　　c.　Exercising

　　　　　　d.　Maintaining approximate weight

　　　　　　e.　Blood pressure

　　　　　　f.　Alcohol consumption

VII. The Health Profile of Seniors

　　A.　Life expectancy is the average number of years of life remaining for a cohort at a particular age.

　　B.　The five leading causes of mortality for seniors are:

　　　　　　a.　Heart disease

　　　　　　b.　Cancer

　　　　　　c.　Stroke

　　　　　　d.　Chronic obstructive pulmonary disease

　　　　　　e.　Pneumonia

　　C.　Morbidity impacts on the quality of life.

　　　1.　Chronic conditions are systemic health problems.

　　　2.　Impairments are deficits in functions of one's sense organs or one's mobility.

　　D.　Health behavior and lifestyle choices are still an important way to improve one's health, even in later life.

TEACHING IDEAS

Lecture Presentation. As a means of introducing the information contained in this chapter, list the five age-groups (i.e., infants and children, etc.) on the chalk board and explain why these five groups are used. Then ask your students to identify what they believe to be the major health problem for the people in each of the groups. With their responses on the board, have the students separate them into personal and/or community health problems. Discuss their answers and indicate why or why not they are correct.

Chapter Wrap-up. After you have presented the content in this chapter, ask the students to create a health profile for the people living in their hometown. Have them write a sentence or two about the primary community health problems in their hometown health for the different age-groups noted in the chapter.

ANNOTATED REFERENCES

APHA & American Academy of Pediatrics. (1992). <u>Caring for our children</u> Washington, D.C.: APHA Publications. This comprehensive text discusses the development and evaluation of the health and safety aspects of family/group day care homes and child care centers. It includes specific guidelines for planning and practical use by the caregiver.

DiClemente, R.J. (1992). <u>Adolescents and AIDS: A generation in jeopardy</u>. Newbury Park, CA: Sage Publishing, Inc. This text studies the AIDS epidemic among adolescents and the behavior that contributes to the spread of the disease. It also discusses programs designed to change behavior, and examines the relationship among adolescents, AIDS, and public policy.

Leach, P. (1994). <u>Children first: What our society must do -and is not doing- for our children today</u>. New York: Alfred A. Knopf. The author argues that Western society is not succeeding in protecting and improving the lives of children. She specifically discusses daycare, discipline, and preschool education, and suggests changes that would improve the treatment of children.

Lee, P.R., & Estes, C.L. (1990). <u>The nation's health</u>, 3rd edition. Boston, MA: Jones and Bartlett Publishers. This text describes the factors that affect the health of Americans. It includes information concerning the health care crisis, issues in health policies for the 1990s, and the future of health care.

Millstein, S., Petersen A., & Nightingale, E. (Eds.). (1993). <u>Promoting the health of adolescents: New directions for the twenty-first century</u>. New York: Oxford University Press. This book focuses on the establishment of healthy lifestyles in adolescents. The social, behavioral, and environmental factors that affect the health behavior are discussed.

ANNOTATED AUDIOVISUALS

BBC-TV Production. <u>Cancer: A genetic disease</u>. Northbrook, IL: Coronet/MTI Film and Video. This video looks at cancer as a genetic and environmental disease. It examines research being conducted on cell growth and eating habits and the records of atom bomb survivors. (26 minute videocassette)

CWI Productions. <u>Our nation's health: A question of choice</u>. Wilton, CT: Author. This video examines changes in diet, exercise, and health monitoring as they affect heart disease. Health care professionals discuss heart disease prevention programs. (59 minute videocassette)

Documentary Production Unit, Dept. of Journalism, University of Illinois. <u>Drinking 101: An introduction to alcohol at the University of Illinois</u>. Urbana, IL: WILL-TV 12. This video addresses the alcohol problem at the University of Illinois which includes alcohol-related deaths, rape, arson, and theft. It examines the effects of student alcoholism and suggests ways to minimize the negative effects of alcohol abuse on campuses.

Sunburst Communications. <u>Fighting back: Teenage depression</u>. Pleasantville, NY: Author. [39 Washington Ave., P.O. Box 40, Pleasantville, NY 10570-0040]. This program focuses on three teenagers and how they experienced and overcame depression. It also suggests ways to get help. (44 minute videocassette)

Words & Music Unlimited. <u>Imagine this</u>. San Diego, CA: Author. Six college students, which have been affected by AIDS, discuss the issue of the disease on college campuses.

CHAPTER 8

Maternal, Infant, and Child Health

CHAPTER SYNOPSIS

This chapter is the first of several in which we discuss the health problems of specific subpopulations: mothers, infants, and children. First, we discuss maternal, then infant, and finally child health issues. Then we review the unique health insurance concerns of this group. Finally, we outline programs that could bring about an improvement in maternal and child health.

CHAPTER OUTLINE

I.   Introduction

    A.   Maternal, infant and child health encompasses the health of women of child-bearing age from pre-pregnancy, through pregnancy, labor and delivery, and the post-partal period.

    B.   It also includes the health of the child prior to birth, through adolescence.

II. Maternal Health

    A.   Maternal mortality rates

        1.   Maternal mortality rates in the U.S. have declined over the past 20 years.

        2.   The maternal mortality rates for black Americans is four times that for white Americans.

    B.   Factors associated with maternal morbidity and mortality

        1.   absence of prenatal care

        2.   teenage pregnancies

III. Infant Health

    A.   Infant mortality rates

        1.   Infant mortality is the death of a child under one year of age.

        2.   Infant mortality rates are the single most important measure of a community's health.

3. Infant mortality rates declined significantly in the U.S. during the period between 1950-1991.

4. A comparison of infant mortality rates of developed nations reveals that America ranks 24th.

5. There is disparity among infant mortality rates of different sub-populations of Americans.

B. Causes of infant mortality

1. Prematurity and low-birth weight

   a. maternal smoking

   b. maternal use of alcohol and other drugs

   c. poverty and minority status

2. Congenital anomalies

3. Sudden infant death syndrome (SIDS)

IV. Child Health

A. Childhood mortality rates

1. The U.S. ranks 20th in childhood mortality

2. Unintentional injuries are the leading cause of death in children under 15 years.

B. Childhood morbidity

1. Unintentional injuries are a leading cause of childhood morbidity.

2. Infectious diseases, such as measles, continue to infect children who are not immunized.

3. Sexually transmitted diseases such as gonorrhea and HIV also cause considerable morbidity in children under 14 years of age.

4. Poor oral health in children can result in nutritional problems.

5. Domestic problems often jeopardize the health of children.

C. Pregnancies in childhood

1. More than one-half million babies are born to girls 15-19 years of age each year.

2. More than 11,000 are babies born to girls under 15 years of age.

3. More than 350,000 children are currently in foster care in the U.S.

V. Health Insurance and Health Care for Women, Infants, and Children

A. Routine pediatric care is out of the financial reach of millions of American families.

B. Two-thirds of those who live in medically underserved areas are children and women of child-bearing age.

VI. Solutions and Programs

A. Prevention of maternal and infant morbidity and mortality

1. Planning families

a. Family planning is determining preferred number and spacing of children and choosing the appropriate means to achieve this preference.

b. Family planning clinics provide a variety of services to assist in family planning.

2. Legalized abortion is controversial

a. Pro-life groups believe abortion is murder.

b. Pro-choice groups believe women have a right to reproductive freedom.

3. Reducing teenage pregnancies

a. Community-based risk reduction programs can successfully reduce teenage pregnancies.

b. Successful risk reduction programs save the community money.

4. Programs that provide prenatal care along with nutritional programs such as the W.I.C. program are successful and save money.

5. Maintaining accurate records of birth defects could reduce the risk and improve access to care.

6. Programs that support SIDS infants can assist families of SIDS victims.

7. Providing supplemental nutrition through the W.I.C. program saves lives, reduces morbidity, and saves money.

B. Prevention of Childhood Morbidity and Mortality

1. Programs that encourage the use of child safety seats, smoke detectors, helmets and life jackets, reduce childhood morbidity and mortality from unintentional injuries.

2. Complete immunization of every child would reduce morbidity from preventable illnesses.

3. Listening to children's advocates can save children's lives.

a. United Nations Children's Fund (UNICEF)

b. Children's Defense Fund

c. American Academy of Pediatrics

4. Accessibility of high quality, affordable child care in America can reduce morbidity and mortality rates for childhren.

TEACHING IDEAS

Interviews. In order to make the information in this chapter more applicable to college-age students, have each student in class interview a young mother. During the interview have your students ask the following questions: 1) What do you see as the greatest health risks for your child(ren) today? 2) What is your greatest health risk? 3) How could the U.S. improve the health care system for mothers, infants, and children? Once the data are collected, pool the responses and compare the results with the content provided in the chapter.

Guest Panel. Invite several mothers to your class (If a large segment of your class is comprised of non-traditional students who are also mothers, randomly select some to sit on the panel). Ask each panel member to share with the class the health concerns they and their children have faced over the years and ask them to offer suggestions on how the health care system in the U.S. could be improved to offer better care for mothers, infants, and children.

ANNOTATED REFERENCES

Christmas, J.J. et al. (1993). Every woman's health: The complete guide to mind and body. (5th ed.). Garden City, NY: Guild America Books. Written by 15 prominent female physicians, this book offers reliable information and sympathetic advice to women of all ages on their total health care. It includes over 900 medical terms, recommended health examinations, generic equivalents to brand name drugs, and health agencies.

Foley, D., Nechas, E., & the editors of *Prevention* magazine. (1993). Women's encyclopedia of health and emotional healing. Emmaus, PA: Rodale Press. This book is a compendium of health problems that women encounter throughout their lives and solutions for the problems. It is scientifically accurate and intended as a reference volume not a medical guide or manual for self-treatment.

Lifshitz, F., Finch, N.M., & Lifshitz, J.Z. (1991). Children's nutrition. Boston, MA: Jones and Bartlett Publishers. This book procures the theories of nutrition to practice better health care of children from conception through adolescence in health and disease. It was written to present accurate information in a straightforward manner to distinguish between the myths and realities of the many nutrition issues that often worry parents and affect children's health and well being.

Sloane, E. (1993). Biology of women. (3rd ed.). Albany, NY: Delmar Publishers Inc. This book is written to provide a comprehensive look at the human female throughout her life span. It presents information on biological sex differentiation, fetal development, and reproductive anatomy. It is concerned with all the events of a woman's reproductive life from menarche to menopause. It also presents information on sexuality, birth control, infertility, pregnancy, sexually transmitted diseases, other health problems, medical examination and other health care.

U. S. Department of Health and Human Services. (1991). Healthy children 2000. (DHHS Publication No. HRSA-A-CH 91-2). Boston, MA: Jones and Bartlett Publishers. This volume is a special compendium of approximately 170 national health promotion and disease prevention objectives affecting mothers, infants, children, adolescents and youth contained in Healthy People 2000, the set of 300 objectives for the nation that was published in September, 1990.

ANNOTATED AUDIOVISUALS

American Academy of Pediatrics. <u>A gift, an obligation</u>. Evanston, IL: Author. [1801 Hinman Ave., Evanston, IL, 60204]. This is a program to inform people of the dangers of childhood diseases and to encourage parents to make sure that they are fully immunized. (30 minute 16 mm film) [Note: This film could also be used with Chapters 3 or 6]

Georgetown University School of Foreign Service. <u>Children at risk</u>. Washington, D.C.: Author. This program studies the health problems, particularly malnutrition and diseases, of the world's children. (30 minute videocassette)

MacNeil/Lehrer Productions. <u>Children at risk</u>. Alexandria, VA: PBS Video. Dr. C. Everett Koop takes a look at the health care system, its problems, and how they affect America's children. The program offers possible solutions to benefit rural and urban children. (58 minute videocassette)

Metropolitan Life Foundation. <u>You can see tomorrow</u>. New York, NY: Author. [Health and Safety Education Division, One Madison Ave., NY, NY, 10010]. This program is a documentary film intended to help teachers and parents to be more aware of their children's health, and to encourage them to take appropriate action when required. The film not only focuses on the prevention and recognition of problems such as vision, hearing, nutrition, infectious diseases and allergies, but also touches on emotional and behavioral issues. (30 minute 16 mm film) [Note: This film could also be used with Chapter 6]

WGBH. <u>Child survival: the silent emergency</u>. Northbrook, IL: Coronet Films & Video. This program examines infant mortality in developing nations and describes a child survival plan developed by UNICEF. (58 minute videocassette)

CHAPTER 9

Community Health and Minorities

CHAPTER SYNOPSIS

The proportion of Americans who belong to a minority group is growing. In 1990, 1 in 5 Americans was a minority group member. Minority groups often bear a heavier burden of disease and other health problems than the general population. In this chapter, we review the disparities in health statistics between various minority groups and the general population. We discuss the causes of these disparities and then suggest three approaches which, if implemented, could eliminate them.

CHAPTER OUTLINE

I. Introduction

    A. Racial, ethnic and cultural diversity is an American strength.

    B. Our population continues to become more diverse.

    C. There are significant disparities in levels of health between the various minorities and the general population.

II. Data Sources and Their Limitations

    A. Classifications of minorities are not completely standardized.

    B. It is necessary to <u>operationalize</u> some minority group definitions in order to discuss health problems of these groups.

III. Americans of Hispanic Origin

    A. Socioeconomic characteristics

        1. There are more than 22 million Hispanic Americans; 87% of Hispanic Americans live in just 10 states.

        2. Hispanics lag behind the general population in education.

        3. Income and employment levels for Hispanics are lower than for non-Hispanic populations.

4. Poverty and lack of education contributes to the poorer health status of Hispanics as a group.

B. Vital statistics

   1. Both birth and fertility rates for Hispanics are higher than those of the overall population.

   2. Years of potential life lost (YPLL) for male Hispanics are higher than for non-Hispanic white Americans.

   3. Crude mortality rates for Hispanics are lower than those for Americans in general.

   4. Infant mortality rates for Hispanic Americans are lower than for the general population.

C. HIV/AIDS in Americans of Hispanic Origin.

   1. For women of child-bearing age, HIV/AIDS rates are higher in Hispanic women than in non-Hispanic white women.

   2. HIV/AIDS rates are higher in children of Hispanic origin than in non-Hispanic white Americans.

IV. Asian/Pacific Islanders

A. Asian/Pacific Islander culture

   1. Culturally, this subpopulation is the most diverse of any of the minority groups.

   2. As a group, Asian/Pacific Islanders share a greater sense of obligation toward their families than do members of other groups.

B. Vital statistics

   1. Birth and fertility rates are higher in Asian/Pacific Islanders than in the general population.

   2. Years of potential lost (YPLL) in this group are the lowest for any sub-population.

   3. Mortality rates for this group are relatively low but the leading causes of death are similar to those of other groups.

   4. Infant mortality rates for Asian/Pacific Islanders are the lowest of any minority in the U.S.

C. Tuberculosis: A community health problem in Asian/Pacific Islanders

   1. Tuberculosis affects racial/ethnic minorities at higher rates than the white population.

   2. Asian/Pacific Islanders have the highest rate of TB of any minority, and one that is 9.9 times higher than the white majority.

V. Black Americans

   A. Understanding the past: the history of blacks in America is one reason why this group continues to be disadvantaged in receiving adequate health care today.

   B. Socioeconomic characteristics

      1. Disparities in socioeconomic status between black and white populations contribute to disparities in health status between the two groups.

      2. Facets of this problem include unemployment, under-employment, under-education and poverty.

   C. Vital statistics

      1. Birth and fertility rates of black Americans are higher than those of the general population.

      2. Life expectancy rates are lower than for other groups.

      3. Years of potential life lost (YPLL) are the highest of any racial or ethnic group in America.

      4. Mortality rates are higher than for other groups.

      5. Leading causes of death are heart disease, stroke, cancer, homicides and legal intervention, and HIV infections.

      6. Infant mortality rates in the black population have declined but remain the highest of any group.

   D. Community health problems of black Americans

      1. Infant mortality

      2. Sickle cell disease

      3. Other noncommunicable health problems

      4. HIV/AIDS

VI. Native Americans

   A. Native Americans share unique beliefs that bind members of this culture together.

   B. Demographic characteristics of Native Americans

      1. Native Americans are likely to be younger, come from larger families and have smaller than average incomes.

      2. They are more likely to be less educated and poorer than members of the general population.

   C. Vital statistics

      1. Birth rates of Native Americans are higher than those of the general population.

2. Their life expectancy is lower than the general population.

3. Years of potential life lost (YPLL) are high, ranking second only to those for black Americans.

4. Mortality rates for this population are lower than those for the general population.

5. Leading causes of death are heart disease, cancer, unintentional injuries, stroke, chronic liver disease and diabetes.

6. Infant mortality rates are very low.

D. The Native Americans and health care

1. The original agency for overseeing Indian Welfare was the Bureau of Indian Affairs.

2. The Indian Health Service, established in 1954, was the first federal agency to address health needs of Native Americans in a comprehensive way.

E. Indian Health Service (IHS)

1. Goal of the IHS is to raise the health status of American Indians and Alaska natives to the highest possible level.

2. The IHS health care system integrates preventive, community and clinical aspects of health care programming.

F. Community health problems of Native Americans

1. Alcohol abuse is a serious problem in Native American communities.

   a. Historical theory

   b. Physiological factors

   c. Social factors

2. Intentional and unintentional injuries are major causes of morbidity and mortality.

   a. Unintentional injuries are the second leading cause of death for Native American males and the third leading cause of death in females.

   b. Homicide and suicide rates in this population are twice those for the general population.

VII. Refugees: The New Immigrants

A. Because America is a prosperous and stable country and because there is turmoil elsewhere, many people come to America from other countries each day seeking a better life.

B. Because newly arrived refugees and other immigrants often have few resources, they put an additional burden on our health care delivery system.

VIII. Solutions to the Community Health Problems of Racial/Ethnic Minorities

    A.   Addressing poverty would reduce many disparities in the health status of different groups of Americans.

    B.   Providing universal access to health care services would improve the health of minorities and narrow the gap in health status between minorities and the general population.

    C.   Empowering people and communities to pursue solutions to their own problems can have a lasting effect on health statistics.

TEACHING IDEAS

Guest Panel. After the material for this chapter has been presented, invite three or four individuals who are either of an ethnic or racial minority to class. Current students from your class may be appropriate. Another resource for contacting these individuals may be through the international student office on campus. Let each panelist provide a little background on his/herself and then let them respond to questions from the class. It may be helpful to ask your students to write questions for the speakers a few days before class so you can sort through them to take out irrelevant and group-like questions.

Interview. Have each student in class interview at least two other individuals of an ethnic or racial group other than his/her own. During the interview have your students ask the following questions: 1) Do you see your race or ethnic origin as being a help or hindrance when it comes to your health? Why or why not? 2) What is your greatest health risk? 3) How could the U.S. improve the health care system to insure access for all? 4) Any other questions the students would like to ask. Once the data are collected have the students share their results and reactions to what they found orally in class.

ANNOTATED REFERENCES

Jackson, J., Chatters, L., & Taylor, R. (Eds.). (1992). Aging in Black America. Newbury Park, CA: Sage Publications, Inc. This source studies aging blacks, their specific circumstances and ability to cope with their changing situations. The information is based on analyses of data from a national survey of the population.

McAdoo, H.P. (Ed.). (1993). Family ethnicity: Strength in diversity. Thousand Oaks, CA: Sage Publications, Inc. This text studies five cultural groups and the issues they face; poverty, inequality, isolation, discrimination, and assimilation versus accommodation. The five groups include: African Americans, Hispanics, Native Americans, Asian Americans, and Muslim Americans.

National Institute of Mental Health. (1991). Mental health services for refugees. Rockville, MD: Department of Health & Human Services. This government publication provides information concerning how to help refugees who are experiencing behavior or mood disorders or adjustment problems.

Stanford, E. & Torres-Gil, F. (Eds.). (1992). Diversity: New approaches to ethnic minority aging. Amityville, NY: Baywood Publishing Co. This monograph focuses on the need for an understanding of the diversity of our aging population and the ideal of eliminating racism and nativism. The text studies future considerations as the aging population becomes more diverse.

Zane, N., Takeuchi, D., & Young, K. (Eds.). (1993). Confronting critical health issues of Asian and Pacific Islander Americans. Thousand Oaks, CA: Sage Publications, Inc. This text looks at health issues and problems specific to Asian and Pacific Islander populations in the United States.

ANNOTATED AUDIOVISUALS

Films for the Humanities & Sciences. AIDS, Teens and Latinos. Princeton, NJ: Author. [P.O. Box 2053, Princeton, NJ 08543-2053]. This program studies factors that contribute to the increased incidence of the HIV virus among Hispanic women, as well as increasing numbers of teenage pregnancies among this same population. (28 minute videocassette)

Films for the Humanities & Sciences. Diabetes and African Americans. Princeton, NJ: Author. [P.O. Box 2053, Princeton, NJ 08543-2053]. Approximately 10% of the African American population have diabetes. This program looks at the causes: genetic factors, obesity, poor diet, lack of exercise, and stress. It explains the disease and its warning signs, and encourages high-risk individuals to get tested. (19 minute videocassette)

Films for the Humanities & Sciences. The culture of poverty. Princeton, NJ: Author. [P.O. Box 2053, Princeton, NJ 08543-2053]. This program shows the problems brought on by poverty that many Latino families experience. Suggestions for breaking the cycle are explored, focusing on reaching and educating Latino children.

Films for the Humanities & Sciences. HB Masters Sickle-Cell Anemia. Princeton, NJ: Author. [P.O. Box 2053, Princeton, NJ 08543-2053]. A character named HB and a teacher explain sickle-cell anemia, a disease common among African Americans. It also suggests how school-age individuals can cope with and manage their disease.

Lupus Foundation of America. Lupus: An issue for the African American community. Columbus, OH: Author. [Marcy Zitron Chapter, 5180 E. Main St., Columbus, OH 43213]. This video discusses Lupus as it affects African American women. It explains the disease, and shows how it affects people who have it. Also offers coping strategies. (28 minute videocassette)

CHAPTER 10

Seniors

CHAPTER SYNOPSIS

The median age of Americans is increasing and is expected to continue to rise for years to come. The aging of the American population presents a variety of socioeconomic and community health problems, including a declining dependency ratio and a growing need for health care services. In this chapter we define terms used to discuss aging and health care, debunk myths about aging, and explain the demographics of aging. We also discuss the unique health care needs of seniors and community efforts to meet these needs.

CHAPTER OUTLINE

I.   Introduction

    A.   Americans are living longer.

    B.   The aging of Americans gives rise to economic, social, political and health care issues.

II. Definitions

    A.   Aged: the state of being old

    B.   Aging: the changes that occur as living things grow older

    C.   Elderly: over 60 years

    D.   Gerontology: study of aging

    E.   Geriatrics: medical practice specializing in treatment of the aged

    F.   Seniors: a preferred term for elderly; a person over 65

III. Myths Surrounding Aging

    A.   Life goes downhill after 65.

    B.   Old people are all the same.

    C.   Old people are lonely and ignored by their families.

    D.   Old people are senile.

E. Old people have a good life.

F. Most old people are sickly.

G. Old people no longer have sexual interest or ability.

H. Most old people end up in nursing homes.

I. Older people are unproductive.

IV. Demography of Aging

   A. Size and growth of the senior population.

      1. The proportion of the population who are seniors has increased throughout the century.

      2. In 1992, 1 in 8 Americans was over the age of 65.

      3. The median age of Americans in 1990 was 33 years and rising.

   B. Factors that affect population size and age.

      1. The fertility rate, the number of births per 1000 women of child-bearing age per year, are declining.

      2. Mortality rates in the United States are declining.

      3. Migration into the United States increases the population.

   C. Dependency (support) and labor-force ratios

      1. The dependency ratio is a comparison of the number of people of working age (20-64 years) to the number not of working age (under 20 or over 64 years).

      2. As the population ages, the total dependency ratio can be expected to decrease.

   D. Other demographic variables of aging

      1. Marital status in seniors depend on one's sex.

         a. Senior men are most likely to be married.

         b. Senior women are most likely to be widowed.

      2. Sixty-nine percent of seniors live with another person; nearly 4 out of 5 seniors who live alone are women.

      3. The vast majority of seniors are white but that the composition is changing.

      4. California and Florida have large senior populations.

      5. The economic status of seniors has improved but remains lower than those of the 25-64 year age group.

6. Housing among seniors is variable.

    a. Twenty-two percent of all households are headed by seniors.

    b. Three-fourths of senior households were owner occupied.

    c. For some seniors housing is a heavy burden.

V. Special Needs of Seniors

    A. Income needs of seniors are generally less than those of younger Americans.

        1. Income reduction accompanies retirement.

            a. Many expenses also decline

            b. Medical expenses often increase

        2. Sources of income

            a. Retirement benefits (including social security and pensions)

            b. Earnings from jobs

            c. Income from assets

            d. Public assistance

            e. Miscellaneous

        3. Twenty-seven percent of seniors are below 150% of poverty line.

    B. Housing needs of seniors are unique.

        1. Housing is important to seniors, not only as shelter, but as a source of continuity.

        2. There is often a need for physical modification of senior housing to accommodate the frailness associated with aging.

        3. Decisions to relocate seniors from independent housing to group housing are usually different and may be stressful for seniors.

        4. Some seniors live in specially designed retirement communities.

        5. A recent innovation in retirement living is the continuing-care retirement community.

    C. Health care needs represent a major issue for seniors.

        1. More than 4 out of 5 seniors live with at least on chronic condition; many have several. These include:

            a. Arthritis

            b. Hypertension

      c.   Hearing impairment

      d.   Heart disease

      e.   Cataracts

      f.   Orthopedic impairments

      g.   Chronic sinusitis

      h.   Diabetes

      i.   Visual impairments

      j.   Varicose veins

2. Seniors are the heaviest users of the health care system.

      a.   More visits to physician

      b.   More hospitalization

      c.   Longer hospital stays

      d.   More dental care

      e.   More eye care

      f.   More money spent on health care services

3. Health care costs for seniors will continue to escalate.

D. Access to transportation is of prime importance for seniors because it enables them to remain independent.

1. Seniors have three levels of transportation needs.

      a.   Those who can use available transportation without help.

      b.   Those who can use available transportation with assistance.

      c.   Those who cannot use currently available transportation and need special services.

2. There are four components to the ideal solution to transportation problems of seniors.

      a.   Fare reductions

      b.   Subsidies to mass transit

      c.   Subsidies for taxis

      d.   Funds to assist senior citizen centers in purchasing specially equipped vehicles.

E. Community facilities and services

    1. <u>Meal service</u> is often available through such programs as meals-on-wheels and congregate meals programs.

    2. <u>Homemaker service</u> enables elderly to remain in their own homes.

    3. <u>Chore and home maintenance service</u> includes yard work, gutter cleaning, and minor plumbing and electrical repair.

    4. <u>Visitor service</u> serves both home bound and institutional seniors.

    5. <u>Adult day care service</u> provides care for seniors who are unable to be left alone all day.

    6. <u>Respite care service</u> allows families who have primary responsibility for a senior to leave their senior in a supervised setting for a short period.

    7. <u>Home health care services</u> are a full range of services including preventive, primary, rehabilitative and therapeutic services provided in the client's home.

    8. <u>Senior centers</u> are facilities where seniors can congregate for fellowship, meals, education and recreation.

    9. There is no limit to the type of services that a community might offer seniors.

F. Personal care

    1. Types of tasks for which seniors might need assistance.

        a. Instrumental tasks, such as housekeeping, transportation and business errands.

        b. Expressive tasks, such as socializing and emotional support.

        c. Cognitive tasks, such as scheduling, reminding and monitoring.

        d. Daily living tasks, such as eating, bathing and dressing.

    2. Types of care givers

        a. Informal care givers are unpaid care givers.

        b. Vare-providers identify and provide care.

        c. Care-managers identify needs and make arrangements for a paid or unpaid care givers who provides services.

TEACHING IDEAS

Field Trip. Make arrangements to take your class to a nursing home or a senior citizen's center. Ask the person in charge to give you a tour of the facility so that the students have a good idea of the services offered. After the tour have your students, either by themselves or in pairs, visit with a senior for approximately a half an hour. During your next class session get the reactions of your students to them either in writing or orally. Also at this time, clear up any misunderstandings your students have and answer their questions.

Guest Panel. After the material for this chapter has been presented, invite three or four seniors to class. If possible try to get one in his/her fifties, one in his/her sixties, and one in his/her seventies or above. You may be able to find volunteers through the senior citizen's center or through the local agency on aging. Let each panelist provide a little background on his/herself including any special health concerns or needs and then let them respond to questions from the class. It may be helpful to ask your students to write questions for the speakers a few days before class so you can sort through them to take out irrelevant questions and group-like questions.

ANNOTATED REFERENCES

Cavanaugh, J.C. (1990). Adult development and aging. Belmont, CA: Wadsworth Publishing Company. This textbook provides a comprehensive overview of gerontology. Specifically, the book presents (1) a comprehensive account of adult development and aging, (2) the theoretical and empirical bases that enable the reader to become educated and a critical consumer of gerontological information, (3) a blend of basic and applied research that demonstrates the range and limitations of current knowledge, and (4) findings from multiple perspectives to show that adult development and aging is an emergent, vibrant, multidisciplinary field.

Christian, J.L., & Grzybowski, J.M. (1993). Biology of aging. St. Louis, MO: Mosby - Year Book, Inc. This textbook was designed for students who will end up working with the elderly as part of their profession. The book provides basic background information on the aging population and the theories of aging. After this introductory material, it provides relevant anatomy and physiology information on each system of the body followed by on how aging affects each system. It concludes with a discussion on the impact of lifestyles on aging. In order to apply the content, the chapters that present a system of the body also contain several case histories.

Digiovanna, A.G. (1994). Human aging: Biological perspectives. New York, NY: McGraw-Hill, Inc. This textbook was written for undergraduate students who have minimal or no science background. The book contains information on the biology of aging via the contributions of the different systems of the body and the relevant anatomy and physiology, and the diseases that affect each system and in turn impact the elderly.

Ferrini, A.F., & Ferrini, R.L. (1993). Health in the later years. (2nd ed.). Madison, WI: Brown & Benchmark Publishers. This book was designed for use in courses in health and aging for upper level undergraduate students. Though the text does include chapters on the biology of aging, it's main focus is on the issues that are associated with the aging process. Therefore, chapters on chronic and acute illness, medication use, medical care, long-term care, sexuality, and death and dying are presented.

Hooyman, N.R., & Kiyak, H.A. (1993). Social gerontology: A multidisciplinary perspective. (3rd ed.). Boston, MA: Allyn and Bacon. This textbook, which is aimed at undergraduate students, has as its primary focus social gerontology. It is comprehensive in nature and examines social aging from biological, physiological, psychological, societal, and social perspectives. It does not cover each of these topics in great detail, but does provide a good overview of all.

ANNOTATED AUDIOVISUALS

American Lung Association. Fight the flu and win. Evans City, PA: Author. [P.O. Box 1036, Evans City, PA 16033]. This program focuses on seniors and their risk of getting the flu. It explains what flu is and who should get a shot. (8 minute videocassette)

Films for the Humanities and Sciences. <u>Ageless America</u>. Princeton, NJ: Author. [P.O. Box 2053, Princeton, NJ 08543-2053]. The process of aging for today's baby boomers is discussed. The program examines views on aging and how and why they have changed. (45 minute videocassette)

Films for the Humanities and Sciences. <u>Aging</u>. Princeton, NJ: Author. [P.O. Box 2053, Princeton, NJ 08543-2053]. The program studies how aging affects various body systems. It also examines how some aging effects can be reversed or slowed down. (28 minute videocassette)

NLN Video. <u>Who will care for an aging America</u>? New York: Author. This program examines the health care needs of aging individuals. Nurses' roles in a variety of settings are also discussed. (25 minute videocassette)

United Cerebral Palsy Associations. <u>When May comes, we'll move to the first floor</u>. Indianapolis, IN: Author. A diary of a young woman with cerebral palsy is shared. Not only are the woman's own frustrations with the disease discussed, but concern about her aging mother who cares for her is also examined. (22 minute videocassette)

CHAPTER 11

Community Mental Health

CHAPTER SYNOPSIS

Mental illness is a major community health issue because of its prevalence and the demands it places on community resources. Over the years, society has tried many approaches to meeting the needs of the mentally ill. Today, communities continue to struggle to provide adequate health and social services to this special, but diverse population. This chapter reviews history of this struggle and elucidates current issues in mental health care including the mentally ill homeless, treatment and social services for the mentally ill, and the federal government's reorganization of its agencies for mental health.

CHAPTER OUTLINE

I.   Introduction

    A.   Mental illness is one of the major issues in community health today.

    B.   Needs and services in mental health are extremely diverse.

    C.   Definitions

        1.   Mental health is the psychological, emotional and social adjustment of a person to the environment.

        2.   Mental disorders are deficiencies in one's psychological resources for dealing with everyday life.

    D.   Classification of mental disorders

        1.   The DSM-III-R published by the American Psychiatric Association represents the best current thinking on classification of mental disorders.

        2.   Mental disorders can be classified by type of onset.

            1.   Mental disorders can be classified by type of onset.

            2.   Mental disorders with onset in adolescence or adulthood.

    E.   Causes of mental disorders include:

        1.   Deficiency at birth

       2.   Physical impairment

       3.   Idiopathic causes

       4.   Environmental factors

       5.   Inherited factors

II.   Mental Illness in America

    A.   Statistical indicators of mental illness

       1.   Between 4 and 5 million Americans are seriously mentally ill.

       2.   Between 15-16% of adults have had at least one episode of a mental disorder in the past 30 days.

       3.   More than 18 of 1000 adults had an episode of serious mental illness in the past year.

    B.   Social indicators of mental illness

       1.   There are nearly 30,000 suicides each year.

       2.   Homicides and suicides are the second and third leading causes of death in those 15-24 years of age.

       3.   In 1990 the divorce rate was nearly half of the marriage rate.

       4.   About four and one-half million women of child-bearing age are current users of illegal drugs.

       5.   There is widespread abuse of alcohol and tobacco in this country.

    C.   Stress: A contemporary mental health problem

       1.   Stress is a normal response to stressors (stress producing stimuli) in our environment.

       2.   Over exposure to high levels of stressors can result in diseases of adaptation such as ulcers, high blood pressure, and impaired immune system function.

       3.   Chronic exposure to stressors can result in mental illness, including alcohol and other drug abuse disorders.

       4.   Entire communities living under stress can respond to social events in a seemingly irrational manner, such as rioting.

III. History of Mental Health Care in America

    A.   Mental health care before World War II

       1.   In early colonial America, the mentally ill were cared for by their families.

       2.   Those without families ended up in poor houses or crude hospitals.

3. In the nineteenth century, moral treatment, based on the theory that mental illness resulted from moral deterioration, was practiced.

   a. Patients were placed in quiet, country settings away from temptations of society and stressors.

   b. Moral treatment was successful as long as there were relatively few patients to treat and patients were a homogeneous lot.

   c. These programs become unsuccessful when facilities were swamped with large numbers of patients at the end of the century.

4. State supported hospitals arose to meet the needs of the growing numbers of mentally ill.

   a. Dorothea Dix was a major proponent of the state hospital system.

   b. The number of state hospitals grew rapidly during the last 25 years of the ninteenth century.

5. The mental hygiene movement arose in the early twentieth century.

   a. Dr. Adolf Meyer championed the idea of early treatment for the mentally ill at special psychopathic hospitals.

   b. Clifford Beers spent a lifetime urging greater efforts to prevent and treat mental illness.

B. Mental health care after World War II

1. Serious federal commitment to the improvement of mental health care began with the passage of the National Mental Health Act of 1946.

2. The National Mental Health Act of 1946 established the National Institutes of Health.

3. Deinstitutionalization, the discharging of mental patients from state hospitals to local communities, began in earnest in the 1950s.

4. New drugs, such as Thorazine, for treating mental illness were another force that propelled deinstitutionalization.

5. Two examples of federal legislation in the 1960s that provided social assistance to the elderly and poor who were mentally ill are:

   a. Community Mental Health Centers Act of 1963

   b. Medicare and Medicaid (1966)

6. The community support movement which began in 1977, is aimed at strengthening community services for the chronically mentally ill.

IV. Mental Health Care in America in the 1990s

A. There is no national policy or program that addresses mental illness.

B. Serious problems remain in mental health care programming at the local level.

C. The aftermath of deinstitutionalization continues to foster social problems in the 1990s.

    1. Homelessness

        a. While estimates vary, approximately 1/3 of all the homeless people are mentally ill.

        b. Many of the chronically ill homeless are young and many of these require frequent hospitalization.

    2. Mental health problems among homeless persons

        a. Homeless have higher rates of communicable diseases, including respiratory, skin, and gastrointestinal illnesses, than the general population.

        b. Homeless suffer more injuries, both intentional and unintentional, than domiciled persons.

        c. Nutritional problems are greater in homeless people.

V. Meeting the Needs of the Mentally Ill

A. Primary prevention of mental illness occurs through voluntary agencies such as the National Mental Health Association and its local affiliates.

B. Secondary prevention, the early detection and rapid diagnosis and treatment, has the following goals and approaches:

    1. Treatment goals

        a. Reduce symptoms

        b. Improve functioning

        c. Strengthen coping skills

        d. Improve behavior

    2. Treatment approaches

        a. <u>Biomedical therapy</u> includes pharmaceutical and electroconvulsive therapies.

        b. <u>Psychotherapy</u> involves face to face interviews with trained therapists.

        c. <u>Behavioral therapy</u> involves the use of biofeedback, stress management and relaxation training to change behavior.

C. Social services intervention involves helping those with mental disorders locate and utilize available social support services necessary for independent living.

D. The dilemma of involuntary commitment and mandatory treatment pits the civil rights of the individual against the rights of the community.

VI. Future Outlook

    A. Federal initiatives for mental health care in the 1990s.

        1. Congress has declared the 1990s as the decade of the brain.

        2. A new federal agency, the Substance Abuse and Mental Health Services Administration (SAMHSA), has been established within the U.S. Public Health Service.

        3. SAMHSA has three centers:

            a. The Center for Substance Abuse Treatment (CSAT)

            b. The Center for Substance Abuse Prevention (CSAP)

            c. The Center for Mental Health Services (CMHS)

    B. The National Alliance for the Mentally Ill advocates for the mentally ill.

TEACHING IDEAS

Guest Speaker. Since stress is prevalent in the college population, invite a representative from the counseling center on campus to your classroom. Have the person speak briefly about stress, its causes, and symptoms. Specifically have him/her talk about college life. Then have him/her talk about how the center handles, step-by-step, a case where stress is suspected.

Writing Assignment and Critique. After you have covered the material contained in this chapter in class, have your students write a one page paper on "What a community can do to help prevent mental illness." Then have your students get together in groups of three to five students. Within the groups, the students should read each others' papers and then decide which response is the best. Then have each group present their choice and have the whole class decide which is the best response.

ANNOTATED REFERENCES

Burr, W. & Klein, S. (1993). Reexamining family stress. Thousand Oaks, CA: Sage Publications, Inc. The authors study different families in stress and discuss various patterns in response to family stress. They also examine the usefulness and harmfulness of coping strategies in various families.

Ghadirian, A. & Lehmann H. (Eds.). (1993). Environment and psychopathology. New York, NY: Springer Publishing Co. Authors in this text study the influence of environmental factors on the mental health of individuals. They discuss a variety of environmental risk factors categorized in three areas: physical factors, social-cultural forces, and catastrophic forces as they relate to mental health problems.

Glenwick, D. & Jason, L. (Eds.). (1993). Promoting health and mental health in children, youth, and families. This text examines issues such as physical and sexual abuse, substance abuse, teenage pregnancy, and childhood accidents. The contents also provide theory and history of mental health in the community.

Greenberg, J. (1993). <u>Comprehensive stress management</u>. Madison, WI: Brown & Benchmark. This is a comprehensive text that covers many aspects of the management of stress. It includes scientific foundations and a definition of stress, life situation and perception interventions, relaxation techniques, physiological arousal and behavior change interventions, and specific applications such as occupational stress, family stress, and stress and the college student.

National Institute of Mental Health. (1991). <u>Caring for people with severe mental disorders: A national plan of research to improve services.</u> Rockville, MD: Department of Health & Human Services. This source is a National Advisory Mental Health Council report suggesting ways to improve services research and research resources in order to improve the care for individuals with severe mental disorder

ANNOTATED AUDIOVISUALS

ABC Distribution Co. <u>Why are they here</u>? New York: Author. This "20-20" segment with Hugh Downs and Barbara Walters studies the problem of incarcerating the mentally ill because of a lack of a better place for these individuals. (16 minute videocassette)

Direct Cinema Limited. <u>Asylum.</u> Los Angeles, CA: Author. This program profiles the history of Saint Elizabeth's Hospital, the national mental institution in Washington, D.C. It begins with the hospital's first patient in 1855, and follows patient growth to 7,000 patients in 1950. The civil rights movement in the 1960s helped reduce the patient population, but how to treat the mentally ill remains controversial. (57 minute videocassette)

Films for the Humanities & Sciences. <u>Schizophrenics in the Streets.</u> Princeton, NJ: Author. [PO Box 2053, Princeton, NJ 08543-2053]. This video investigates the quick release of patients from psychiatric facilities. As a result, large numbers of mentally ill individuals are out in society, some living and dying in the streets. The program calls this problem a "scandal" that must be addressed. (28 minute videocassette)

Films for the Humanities & Sciences. <u>Schizophrenia: The voices within/The community without</u>. Princeton, NJ: Author. This program shows the nature of the disease schizophrenia by profiling former Green Bay Packer, Lionel Aldridge, who suffered from the disease. Experts discuss symptoms, treatment, and possible causes. The video then looks at deinstitutionalization of mental patients and the struggle many of them have without aftercare or support from the community. (19 minute videocassette)

WNET/Thirteen. <u>Backwards to back streets</u>. New York: Video Dub. The video shows what happens to mentally ill individuals who are discharged prematurely from hospitals. Also shown are several community health care services that are helping and/or not helping these patients. (59 minute videocassette)

CHAPTER 12

Abuse of Alcohol and Other Drugs

CHAPTER SYNOPSIS

The abuse of alcohol and other drugs is a major community health problem, costing thousands of lives, billions of dollars and untolled anguish each year. In this chapter, we review dimensions of the drug problem in the United States, its causes, and federal, state and local efforts to resolve it. These efforts involve programs to reduce both the supply and demand for drugs.

CHAPTER OUTLINE

I. Introduction

    A. Scope of the problem.

        1. The annual economic loss attributable to drug use in the United States is estimated at $177 billion.

        2. One-third of all high school seniors and college students reported taking at least one illicit drug in the past year.

        3. Marijuana is the number one illicit drug; 14% of high school seniors and college students reported use of marijuana in the past 30 days in 1990.

        4. Use of most illicit drugs has declined in recent years.

        5. Use of alcohol and tobacco has remained about the same in recent years despite efforts to reduce their use.

        6. Misuse of over-the-counter and prescription drugs is substantial.

    B. Definitions

        1. A drug is a substance, other than food or vitamins, that upon entering the body in small amounts, alters one's physical, mental or emotional state.

        2. A psychoactive drug is one that affects the central nervous system.

        3. Drug misuse is the inappropriate use of over-the-counter or prescription drugs.

        4. Drug abuse can be defined in various ways.

            a. The taking of a drug for non-medically approved purposes.

        b.   The continued use of a legal drug with the knowledge that it is hazardous to one's health (cigarette smoking).

        c.   The use of any illegal drug.

    5.   Drug dependence can be psychological, physical or both.

        a.   Psychological dependence is characterized by the strong desire to continue the use of a drug.

        b.   Physical dependence is said to have occurred when discontinuation of drug use results in clinical illness.

II.   Factors that Contribute to the Abuse of Alcohol, Tobacco or Other Drugs

    A.   Inherited risk factors

        1.   There is evidence that at least some types of alcoholism are inherited.

        2.   The heritability of susceptibility to other drugs is still under investigation.

    B.   Environmental risk factors

        1.   Personal factors, factors that relate to the individual, include personality traits such as impulsiveness, depressive mood or personality disturbances.

        2.   Home and family life factors that contribute to drug problems include dysfunctional family dynamics, negative family events and unhealthy family attitudes toward drug use.

        3.   Other family influences are those that result in the failure to develop interpersonal skills and build up self-esteem.

        4.   School and peer group factors include one's school environment, one's peers and perceptions of peer drug use.

        5.   Sociocultural aspects of one's environment can contribute to drug use. Examples include availability of drugs, number and quality of police, and the availability of jobs and recreation facilities.

III. Types of Drugs Abused

    A.   Legal drugs

        1.   Alcohol

            a.   By almost any measure, alcohol is America's number one drug problem.

            b.   More Americans drink alcohol than use any other psychoactive drugs.

            c.   Thirty-two percent of high school seniors and 41% of college students reported having 5 or more drinks in a row at least once in the past two weeks.

            d.   Problem drinkers are those for whom alcohol use results in personal, financial, social or legal problems.

     e.   Alcoholics are those who have impaired control over their drinking, distortions in thinking about alcohol and physical dependence upon alcohol.

  2. Nicotine

     a.   Nicotine use occurs in the form of cigarette, cigar and pipe smoking and in the use of chewing tobacco and snuff.

     b.   Cigarettes are smoked daily by 19% of high school seniors.

     c.   It has been estimated that cigarette smoking causes approximately 400,000 deaths and costs $52 billion annually in the United States.

     d.   Smokers' habits affect nonsmokers through environmental tobacco smoke.

     e.   Smokeless tobacco use is not a safe alternative to smoking.

  3. Over-the-counter (OTC) drugs

     a.   Over-the-counter drugs are those that can be purchased without a doctor's prescription.

     b.   Misuse of OTC drugs is very common

     c.   Most OTC drugs provide only symptomatic relief, not a cure.

  4. Prescription drugs

     a.   Prescription drugs can only be purchased with a physician's written instructions.

     b.   Prescription drugs are usually stronger or more concentrated than over-the-counter drugs.

     c.   There is greater risk for abuse for certain psychoactive prescription drugs, than for OTC drugs.

     d.   Misuse of prescription antibiotics can lead to the formation of drug resistant strains of disease causing bacteria.

B. Illicit (illegal) drugs are those that cannot be cultivated, manufactured, bought, sold or used within the confines of the law.

  1. Marijuana, a product of the hemp plant, cannabis sativa, is the most abused illicit drug in the United States.

     a.   Marijuana use in college students has declined from 34% in 1980 to 14% in 1990.

     b.   Marijuana has both acute and chronic affects upon health.

  2. Opium, morphine and heroin are derivatives of the oriental poppy plant and are classified as narcotics.

     a.   Narcotics numb the senses and reduce pain.

b. There are between 1/2 to 1 million heroin addicts in the U.S.

c. Narcotics produce tolerance and physical dependence.

d. Injection narcotic users are at high risk for becoming infected with HIV and for infecting others with HIV.

3. Cocaine is a potent stimulant that occurs in leaves of the coca plant of South America.

   a. Hallucinogens are drugs that produce hallucinations and synesthesia.

      i. LSD

      ii. Mescaline

      iii. Psilocybin

   b. Designer drugs are drugs prepared illegally by amateur chemists who have altered their chemical structures to evade law enforcement.

      i. Fentanyl and related chemicals

      ii. MPPP

      iii. MDMA and related chemicals

      iv. PCP and related chemicals

   c. Stimulants increase the activity of the central nervous system.

      i. Amphetamine

      ii. Methamphetamine

      iii. Methcathinone

   d. Depressants decrease the activity of the central nervous system.

      i. Barbiturates

      ii. Benzodiazepines

      iii. Methaqualone

   e. Anabolic drugs are protein building drugs, that are sometimes abused by those who wish a short cut to increasing muscle size.

   f. Inhalants are psychoactive, breathable substances often abused by youth.

IV. Prevention and Control of Drug Abuse

   A. Levels of prevention

      1. Primary prevention programs are aimed at those who never used drugs.

2. Secondary prevention programs seek to reach those who have begun drug use but are not chronic drug abusers.

3. Tertiary prevention programs are designed to provide treatment for abuse and aftercare, including relapse prevention programs.

B. Official agencies and programs

1. The 1993 Federal drug control budget was $12.7 billion, a seven-fold increase over the 1981 budget.

   a. Department of Justice (DOJ) has the largest budget to fight drug abuse; funds are used for law enforcement; prisons, and other aspects of the justice system.

      i. The Drug Enforcement Agency (DEA) is the lead agency in the government's war on drugs.

      ii. The Federal Bureau of Investigation (FBI) investigates drug related crimes.

      iii. The Immigration and Naturalization Service (INS) deports alien drug traffickers.

   b. Department of Treasury

      i. U.S. Customs Service patrols our borders

      ii. The Internal Revenue Service (IRS) targets money laundering.

      iii. The Bureau of Alcohol, Tobacco and Firearms (ATF) regulates alcohol and tobacco.

   c. Department of Health and Human Services (DHHS) views drug abuse as a lifestyle problem for which the solution is health promotion and research.

      i. Primary prevention includes education, automatic protection and regulation.

      ii. Secondary prevention includes rapid diagnosis and intervention with treatment.

      iii. The Substance Abuse and Mental Health Services Administration (SAMHSA) is the education training and services agency for the federal government.

      iv. The National Institute of Drug Abuse (NIDA) is the lead federal research agency.

      v. The Food and Drug Administration (FDA) is the federal regulatory agency for legal drugs.

2. State and regional agencies and programs are aimed at assisting local communities in solving their drug problems.

   a. State government can influence the outcome of drug wars through advocacy, administrative aid and legislation.

67

        b.   Regional coordination offices provide a link between state and local efforts.

   3.   Local agencies and programs

        a.   Local coordination council (LCC) are made up of citizen representation from diverse backgrounds.

        b.   Community-based drug education programs can be sponsored by any local institution or organization.

        c.   School-based drug education programs include employee assistance programs (EAP).

   4.   Unofficial agencies and programs

        a.   Mothers Against Drunk Drivers

        b.   Students Against Driving Drunk

        c.   Alcoholics Anonymous

        d.   Narcotics Anonymous

        e.   American Cancer Society

TEACHING IDEAS

Guest Speaker. Invite the Dean of Students from your college/university into your classroom. Ask him/her to give an overview of the drug problem on your campus. Have the dean talk about the process a student must go through when caught abusing drugs and the consequences of abusing drugs on your campus. Also ask him/her to offer his/her suggestions to the problem.

Class Debate. After you have presented the material contained in this chapter, divide the class in half to debate the issue of whether or not marijuana should be legalized. Have each side research the issue and have them examine it from a community health perspective not a personal health one. In other words, what are the pros and cons for a community to legalize this drug?

ANNOTATED REFERENCES

Avis, H. (1993). Drugs and life. Madison, WI: Brown & Benchmark. This is a comprehensive text that begins with an introduction to drugs, the pharmacology of drug action, and the physiology related to drug use. The author then discusses the drug classifications as well as over-the-counter and prescription medicine. The last several chapters contain information about drugs and the law, treatment, drug education, and prevention.

Carroll, C.R. (1993). Drugs in modern society. (3rd ed.). Madison, WI: Brown & Benchmark Publishers. This textbook was designed for use in drug education courses for students from a variety of disciplines. It is a comprehensive text with 14 chapters divided into six sections; introduction, depressants, stimulants, mind-expanding euphoriants, medicines, and prevention of drug abuse.

Meeks, L., Heit, P., & Page R. (1994). Drugs, alcohol, and tobacco. Blacklick, OH: Meeks Heit Publishing Co. This text provides factual information about drugs and drug use, offers an approach for reducing the risk of drug abuse and violence, suggests life skills for well-being and resiliency, and includes skills for good decision making and resistance to drug use and abuse. The authors also offer a variety of teaching strategies.

Pinger, R.R., Payne, W.A., Hahn, D.B., & Hahn, E.J. (1995). Drugs: issues for today. (2nd ed.) St. Louis, MO: Mosby - Year Book, Inc. This textbook, which has been written for use in introductory drug courses for students who have limited background in the life sciences, presents information on the nature of drugs and the issues that surround drug abuse. This second edition includes 17 chapters on drug use, misuse and abuse, impact of drugs on the body, and the prevention and control of drug abuse. There are individual chapters on over-the-counter drugs, prescription drugs, tobacco, alcohol, steroids, stimulants, narcotics, and other groups of controlled substances.

Witters, W., Venturelli, P., & Hanson, G. (1992). Drugs and society. Boston, MA: Jones and Bartlett Publishers. The authors examine the social, economic, and political problems of substance abuse and how they influence society locally, nationally, and internationally. The text also includes drug use and misuse as it affects families, the workplace, neighborhoods, communities, schools, and religious institutions.

ANNOTATED AUDIOVISUALS

Canadian Broadcasting Corporation. Dealing with drugs. New York, NY: Filmakers Library. [124 East 40th St., New York, NY 10016]. This program describes drug abuse as a health problem, not a legal problem. It shows how four major cities deals with drug abuse; New York, Toronto, Amsterdam, and London. The video also suggests new approaches in tackling the problem of drug abuse. (94 minute videocassette)

Films for the Humanities & Sciences. The Drug We Drink. Princeton, NJ. Author. [P. O. Box 2053, Princeton, NJ 08543-2053]. This production offers reasons why people drink, explains the effects of alcohol on the body, and suggests guidelines for maximum alcohol consumption.

Learning Multi-Systems, Inc. Community-wide drug prevention program. Madison, WI: Author. [320 Holtzman Rd., Madison, WI 53713]. Jim Crowley, an authority on adolescents, discusses adolescent alcohol and other drug use and how communities can respond to these problems. A three part series consisting of: Mobilizing your community (31 minute videocassette), Basic guidelines for effective programs (27 minute videocassette), and Helpful programs.

Stanford Center for Research in Disease Prevention. Prevention of alcohol problems. Palo Alto, CA: Author. This program shows the main points of a four hour alcohol abuse workshop. Included are alcohol advertising, the development of community-based programs, and examples of successful interventions. (90 minute videocassette)

WETA-TV. Drinking and driving: the toll, the tears. Washington, D.C.: Author. This Phil Donahue program explores how a drunken driver changed people's lives. Individuals share their stories from a home, a prison, a church, a hospital, and a cemetery. (58 minute videocassette) Note: This videocassette could also be used for Chapter 17.

UNIT III

HEALTH CARE DELIVERY

CHAPTER 13

Health Care System: Structure

CHAPTER SYNOPSIS

In this chapter we discuss America's health care delivery system. First, we briefly review the evolution of health care in the United States over the past 150 years. We then discuss the spectrum of health care delivery, defining the various types of care provided. This is followed by a description of the kinds of health care providers and, finally, by an outline of kinds of facilities in which health care delivery takes place.

CHAPTER OUTLINE

I. Introduction

    A. Health care in the United States is delivered by a variety of providers practicing in an array of settings.

    B. The health care delivery system in the United States includes a haphazard conglomeration of health care providers, facilities, agencies and programs.

II. A Brief History of Health Care Delivery in the United States

    A. Before 1850, health care was often delivered in the patient's home.

    B. Between 1850-1900, medical care progressively moved into doctors' offices and hospitals.

    C. By the beginning of the twentieth Century, scientific discoveries had begun to be reflected in new medical procedures and instruments and improved medical practice.

    D. Following World War II, the rate of new hospital construction accelerated.

    E. Better hospitals, equipment and drugs resulted in escalating costs of treatment.

    F. Rising costs of medical care in the 1950s and 1960s led to an increased interest in health insurance and the growth of the third party payment system.

    G. The mushrooming of the third party payment system fueled increases in medical costs.

    H. By the early 1960s, it had become apparent that the fruits of remarkable medical advances were not reaching large portions of the population, especially the poor and elderly.

I. Medicare and Medicaid were authorized to assist the elderly and the poor to participate in health care.

J. The infusion of federal dollars into the health care system further accelerated the rising costs of health care.

K. Between the 1960s and the 1990s, numerous federal attempts to reduce health care costs through better planning failed.

L. Health care costs by the middle of the 1990s were equal to 14% of the nation's GNP.

III. The Spectrum of Health Care Delivery

   A. <u>Preventive Care</u> is health care aimed at keeping healthy people healthy.

      1. Education is a primary component of preventive care.

      2. Preventive care is practiced by school nurses, nutritionists, health educators and doctors.

      3. Preventive care takes place at home, in schools, in well clinics, fitness programs, family planning clinics and doctors' and dentists' offices.

   B. <u>Primary care</u> is front line care that is comprehensive and person centered.

      1. A central component of primary care is the physical examination.

      2. Those who provide primary care are family practice physicians, dentists, pediatric nurse practitioners, nurses and allied health professionals.

      3. Primary care is given in clinics, doctors' offices, dentists' offices and other out-patient facilities.

      4. Other primary health services are taken for granted in the United States.

         a. Safe and adequate food supply

         b. Clean water

         c. Control of communicable diseases

         d. Immunizations

   C. <u>Secondary care</u> is acute care.

      1. Examples are intense or elaborate diagnosis and treatment, such as setting a broken bone or treating a gonorrhea infection.

      2. This type of care is usually provided by a physician.

      3. This type of care is usually provided in emergency rooms or free standing clinics.

   D. <u>Tertiary care</u> is specialized care.

1. Tertiary care includes treatments for heart disease and cancer of complex surgeries.

2. This type of care is provided by a physician who is a specialist.

3. Tertiary care usually takes place in a large hospital with trained staff.

E. Restorative care is recovery and rehabilitative care.

1. Restorative care includes care after surgery, stroke or cancer treatment.

2. This type of care may be provided by a variety of nurses and allied health personnel.

3. Restorative care is often provided in rehabilitation units of large hospitals or in nursing homes, halfway houses and private homes.

F. Continuing care is long-term health care.

1. This type of care is for chronic health problems, physical or mental, including but not limited to those associated with old age.

2. Continuing care is often provided by nurses and other allied health personnel.

3. The settings for continuing care are nursing homes, state hospitals, halfway houses, and private residences.

IV. Types of Health Care Providers

A. In 1991, an estimated 9.8 million people, 8% of all employed civilians, worked in the health service industry.

1. This number is growing more rapidly than employment in general.

2. Growth is expected to continue.

3. Half of all health care workers are employed in hospitals, 17% in nursing homes and 12% in physicians offices.

4. There are more than 200 different careers in the health care industry.

B. Independent providers have legal authority to treat any health problem.

1. Allopathic and osteopathic providers include medical physicians and osteopathic physicians.

   a. Allopathic providers are those whose specific remedies often include drugs or medication that produce different effects than those of the disease.

   b. Osteopathic providers are graduates from schools of osteopathy and are licensed to practice in all states and the District of Columbia upon passing the respective state's medical examination.

2. Nonallopathic providers are non-traditional health practitioners.

   a. This group includes chiropractors, acupuncturists, naturopaths, homeopaths and naparapaths.

b. Chiropractors provide care based on the premise that health problems arise from misalignments of vertebrae.

3. Limited care providers

   a. Limited health care providers have advanced training in a health specialty and are licensed to practice it.

   b. Examples are dentists, optometrists, podiatrists and psychologists.

4. Nurses

   a. Nursing has a long-standing tradition.

   b. There are 3-4 million nurses in the United States.

   c. Training and education in nursing vary.

      i. Licensed practical nurses (LPN) and licensed vocational nurses (LVN) complete 1-2 years of vocational training and are licensed to carry out non-technical duties under the supervision of doctors and registered nurses.

      ii. Registered nurses (RN) have completed associate or baccalaureate degrees in nursing and have passed a state licensing (registration) exam.

      iii. Technical nurses are registered nurses that hold an associate degree (2 years).

      iv. Professional nurses are registered nurses that hold a baccalaureate degree (4 years).

   d. Specialized training in nursing beyond four years is becoming more common.

      i. Master's degrees

      ii. Doctorate degrees

5. Allied health care professionals comprise many professionals who perform tasks in the health care industry.

   a. Examples are dietitians, physical therapists, medical technologists, medical records keepers, emergency medical technicians, speech therapists, etc.

   b. Many of these professionals will be in high demand in the future.

6. Public health professionals facilitate public health work.

   a. Examples are environmental health workers, public health administrators, epidemiologists, health educators, and biostatisticians.

   b. These professionals usually have advanced education and training.

V. Health Care Facilities

A. Doctors' offices are facilities privately owned by independent practitioners in which health care is delivered.

B. Medical clinics are facilities that are privately owned by two or more physicians or by the public in which health care or medical treatment is delivered.

C. Clinics vary in size from small (with two or three physicians) to very large (Mayo Clinic).

D. Hospitals are public, private, or governmental facilities in which secondary (acute) and tertiary (special) medical care are provided.

    1. Private, proprietary hospitals are owned as a business for the purpose of making a profit.

    2. Governmental hospitals are publicly owned hospitals. Examples include:

        a. Federal: Veterans, Army, Navy, etc.

        b. State: state owned mental hospitals

        c. Local: county or city owned hospitals

    3. Voluntary (independent) hospitals are nonprofit hospitals administered by religious, fraternal, community, or other charitable groups. These hospitals, as a group, provide the most beds in the United States.

E. Rehabilitation centers are health care facilities that provide services aimed at restoring functions lost because of injury, disease, surgery, or other treatment.

F. Continuing care facilities provide long-term, chronic, respite and hospice care.

    1. Examples include nursing homes, mental hospitals, halfway houses and group homes.

    2. This is a growth area in health care.

TEACHING IDEAS

Newspaper Clippings. Prior to presenting the content of this chapter, scan your local newspaper looking for articles that are related to health care delivery. Cut the articles out of the paper and have them made into overhead transparencies. After presenting the information on the spectrum of health care, show the transparencies to the students. Ask them to identify where the information fits into the spectrum of care and ask them to defend their response based upon information presented in the text or class.

Writing Assignment. This activity could be conducted at the beginning or end of the lesson that covers the content in this chapter. Have the students identify what they think is the number one health care problem in their hometown, then have them defend their response. Have several students share their response with the rest of the class and have the other students either agree or disagree with the rationale. If the activity is conducted at the beginning of the class, it can be used as a springboard for the rest of the class time. If it is used at the end of the class, students can be asked to defend their response based on the information presented in text.

ANNOTATED REFERENCES

Jonas, S. (1992). <u>An introduction to the United States health care system</u> (3rd ed.). New York: Springer Publishing Company. This text provides a brief overview of the varied components of our health care system. The author emphasizes principles, structure, and concerns.

Kovner, A. (1990). <u>Health care delivery in the United States.</u> New York: Springer Publishing Company. This text examines a variety of issues: nursing, ambulatory care, hospitals, long term care, mental health services, technology assessment, and ethics.

Reagan, M. (1992). <u>Curing the crisis: Options for America's health care</u>. Boulder, CO: Westview Press. This text studies the current status of health care in the U.S., discussing HMOs, preferred provider organizations, exclusive provider organizations, and combination programs. It also discusses the current problems, explores options, and offers suggestions for a better plan. Also appropriate for Chapter 14.

Stanfield, P. (1990). <u>Introduction to the health professions</u> (2nd ed.). Boston, MA: Jones and Bartlett Publishers. This is a good source for students pursuing a career in the field of health. It provides information for over sixty health related careers and suggests additional sources for more specific information.

The White House Domestic Policy Council. (1993). <u>The Presidents's Health Security Plan</u>. New York: Times Books. This text is the Clinton administration's draft report on health care reform. It contains ideas for addressing the issues of the health-care crisis advocated by President Clinton and Hillary Rodham Clinton.

ANNOTATED AUDIOVISUALS

Films for the Humanities & Sciences. <u>Home care.</u> Princeton, NJ.: Author. [P. O. Box 2053, Princeton, NJ: 08543-2053]. This video looks at the reasons for the growth of home care, the advantages to the patient and the family, and the technology available to make home care possible. (19 minute videocassette)

Films for the Humanities & Sciences. <u>Nursing: A medical emergency.</u> Princeton, NJ: Author. [P. O. Box 2053, Princeton, NJ: 08543-2053]. This program looks at the role of nurses as they care for and treat patients. It compares the skills necessary today for successful nurses to the skills needed in previous years. The video also addresses the nursing shortage and what is being done about it. (19 minute videocassette)

NLN Video. <u>The power of nursing</u>. New York: Author. The Chief Executive Officer of the National League for Nursing interviews three women who were staff nurses and became national leaders in the field of nursing and medical care. They discuss the varied roles of nurses, how they can attain social and political power, and how they can influence health care reform. (25 minute, 37 second videocassette)

UNICEF. <u>The Bamako initiative in action</u>. New York: Author. The video examines the Bamako Initiative, a successful, new approach to primary health care being implemented in a majority of African countries. (35 minute videocassette)

WGBH. <u>The health quarterly</u> (<u>My job, my health</u>, <u>An answer from government</u>, <u>The AIDS report: Decade of the virus</u>). Boston, MA.: Author. [Off-air licensing rights through PBS Video]. This three part television report discusses the status of public health in the United States, looks at the health care system-cost and insurance, and examines the status of the AIDS epidemic. (31 minute, 13 minute, 12 minute videocassettes)

CHAPTER 14

Health Care System: Function

CHAPTER SYNOPSIS

In this chapter, the second on the health care system, we describe how people obtain health care services, how these services are paid for and by whom. We also discuss two important shortcomings of the current system, access and cost, and review possible alternative systems.

CHAPTER OUTLINE

I.   Introduction

    A.   The health care services available in America are among the best in the world.

    B.   Not all Americans have access to these services.

II. Gaining Access to and Paying for Health Care in America

    A.   Access to health care

        1.   Only 86% of Americans have access to the full spectrum of health care.

        2.   While almost all Americans have access to acute (emergency) care, many do not have access to primary care.

        3.   Factors that limit access to health care

            a.   Lack of health insurance

            b.   Inadequate insurance

            c.   Poverty

    B.   Paying for health care

        1.   Health care constitutes America's single largest expenditure (larger than defense).

        2.   America annually spends $2,900 per person for health care.

        3.   Payments for the health care bill come from four sources.

            a.   Direct or out-of-pocket payments

b. Third party payments

 i. Private insurance

 ii. Public funds : Medicare, Medicaid, military

 iii. Private philanthropy

4. Important terms

 a. A <u>fee-for-service system</u> is one in which a service is provided, for example, medical care, in return for which a fee is paid.

 b. A system of <u>third party payments</u> is one in which a fee for service is paid by a third party, an insurance company or government agency, which has collected the funds as insurance premiums or taxes.

II. Health Insurance

A. Health insurance is a risk and cost spreading process.

 1. People at higher risk are sometimes required to pay higher premiums.

 2. People with preexisting conditions may have to pay more, or must carry an exclusion.

B. A health insurance policy is a written agreement between a private company and an individual in which the company agrees to pay for certain health care costs in return for regular periodic payments by the individual to the company (premiums).

 1. A self-insured organization is one that pays the health care costs of its employees with premiums collected from them plus its own contributions.

 2. Health insurance cost in the United States--1992

  a. The average cost per employee for health insurance in 1992 was $5,000.

  b. The annual increase is about 15% per year.

 3. Types of health care coverage. Most policies provide for:

  a. Hospitalization

  b. Surgical procedures

  c. Regular medical costs

  d. Major medical costs

  e. Dental services

  f. Disability payments

IV. Governmental Health Insurance

A. The federal government does not provide health insurance for all citizens.

B. It does provide insurance for two specific populations: the elderly and the poor.

    1. Medicare is health insurance for those 65 years of age and older.

        a. It is administered by the Health Care Financing Administration (HCFA).

        b. It consists of part A, Hospital Insurance and part B, Medical Insurance.

        c. Part A is mandatory; part B is optional and available at an additional charge.

        d. Medicare uses a prospective pricing system in which hospitals are paid a predetermined amount of money based on the specific diagnosis.

    2. Medicaid is health insurance for the poor.

        a. Eligibility for the programs is determined by each state.

        b. There are no age requirements.

        c. Medicaid is a noncontributory program.

V. Supplemental Medicare Coverage

A. Medigap policies cover deductibles, co-insurance and other out-of-pocket expenses incurred by Medicare patients.

B. Medigap programs are now regulated by the federal government.

C. Optional supplemental insurance is available on the private market for non-medicare recipients.

D. Long-term care insurance designed to pay for long-term nursing home care is currently a popular type of supplemental insurance.

VI. Alternatives to the Current System

A. Existing alternatives to the traditional fee-for-service system include health maintenance organizations, national health insurance, and a variety of other health care plans.

    1. Health maintenance organizations combine health care insurance coverage and the delivery of medical services into one package. Members pay monthly fees and in return receive all the health care they need.

        a. In staff model HMOs, salaried physicians provide medical services into one package. Members pay monthly fees and in return receive all the health care they need.

        b. In the group model HMOs, a physicians' group practice contracts with an HMO to provide care to members, but they may also see other patients who are not HMO members.

        c. In the network model HMO, two or more group practices contract with an HMO to provide care for HMO members, while also seeing other patients.

d.   In the <u>independent practice association model</u>, individual physicians contract with an HMO to provide care for HMO members and are paid a set amount for each enrollee. These physicians may also see other patients.

2.   Preferred provider organizations (PPOs) operate still differently.

   a.   PPOs approach a provider and contract with that provider to provide dental services at a discount price to all individuals covered in the PPO's plan.

   b.   Patients can choose another provider but must pay the difference in the cost of services between their chosen provider and the preferred provider.

3.   Exclusive provider organizations (EPOs) are like PPOs except participants must use the EPOs providers and hospitals or else pay the entire bill themselves.

4.   Ambulatory care centers and surgical centers are fee-for-service facilities that are alternatives to the out-patient and emergency room facilities of major hospitals.

   a.   These sites are an efficient alternative for acute care.

   b.   These sites maintain transfer agreements with nearby, full service hospitals.

B.   Innovative programs

1.   Many hospitals have developed new programs in order to compete with ambulatory care and surgical centers.

   a.   Sick child care

   b.   Sick minor care

2.   National health insurance implies a system in which the federal government would ensure the availability of health care services for all people. These services would be paid for by tax dollars.

   a.   Most countries have such systems.

   b.   Congress is considering such a plan this year.

   c.   Clinton Health Care Plan has six points

      i.   Security

      ii.   Cost control

      iii.   Quality

      iv.   Access

      v.   Efficiency

      vi.   Accountability

3.   Description of the Canadian health care system

82

a. The Canadian plan addresses the problem of universal access to health care first and cost second, that is, each province must assure that all residents have access to medical care.

b. Residents have care available to them when they travel to other provinces.

c. Cost is paid by the Canadian government, 30-40%, by private sources, 25%, and by the province, the remainder.

d. Physicians are independent providers.

e. As a result, Canadians spend much less on health care than Americans.

f. There is greater emphasis on prevention and less emphasis on specialized care.

4. The Oregon health plan

a. The Oregon plan addresses <u>cost</u> primarily, and access secondarily.

b. The Oregon plan is based upon the premise that there are finite number of dollars spent on health care in Oregon, and that high priority procedures are to be paid for first with lower priority procedures reimbursed if funds are available.

c. Everyone was consulted in ranking the priority of health care procedures.

d. The state of Oregon was required to obtain a special waiver from the federal government to implement its plan.

e. Many are watching Oregon for indication of success or failure.

TEACHING IDEAS

Analysis of Health Insurance Policy. To help students understand the terminology used in health insurance policies, obtain a copy of the health insurance policy offered to students on your campus. Then after presenting the material in this chapter, read aloud the important portions of the policy and ask students for their interpretation of what you read.

Class Debate. After you have presented the material contained in this chapter, divide the class in half to debate the issue of whether or not health care should be a right or a privilege. Give each side 20 minutes to brainstorm issues and prepare their case. Then give each side 15 minutes to present their side. After the debate, have the students vote on the issue. Conclude by having the students offer solutions to providing care for all.

ANNOTATED REFERENCES

Butler, P. (1988). <u>Too poor to be sick: Access to medical care for the uninsured.</u> Washington, D.C.: American Public Health Association. The author describes the problem of the millions of Americans who lack access to medical care. She offers reasons why current programs are inadequate and suggests possible solutions.

Moon, M. (1993). <u>Medicare now and in the future</u>. Lanham, MD: Urban Institute Press. The author studies the development of the Medicare program over the last twenty-five years and suggests what kinds of changes may emerge. She looks at changes that have been made and changes that have been proposed. The author also makes recommendations.

Navarro, V. (1993). <u>Dangerous to your health: Capitalism in health care</u>. New York: Monthly Review Press. The author examines the United States health care system and compares it with the programs of other Western nations. He focuses on the issue of "class" and criticizes the dominant classes for protecting their own interests and making medical care more difficult to obtain for the working classes.

Navarro, V. (Ed.). (1992). <u>Why the United States does not have a national health program</u>. Amityville, NY: Baywood Publishing Company. Authors in this text study the state of health care in the United States and describe it as "costly and inefficient." The text contains sixteen essays published in the <u>International Journal of Health Services</u>. The authors advocate and suggest a plan for national health care coverage.

Rowland, D., Feder, J., & Salganicoff, A. (Eds.). (1993). <u>Medicaid financing crisis: Balancing responsibilities, priorities, and dollars</u>. Waldorf, MD: AAAS Books. This publication contains seven papers commissioned by the Kaiser Commission. The papers study the causes of spending growth in the Medicaid crisis, examine Medicaid reforms, look at changes in fiscal responsibility by the federal and state governments, and evaluate program management.

ANNOTATED AUDIOVISUALS

CBS News. <u>The Oregon plan</u>. South Burlington, VT: Ambrose Video Pub. This video is from a television broadcast of 60 Minutes with Steve Kroft. It looks at the Oregon Health Care Plan that provides basic health care for Oregon residents and promotes and emphasizes preventive care. The program also discusses some of the plan's problems. (14 minute, 47 second videocassette)

Filmaker's Library. <u>Borderline medicine</u>. New York: Author. [124 East 40th St., New York, NY 10016]. The program compares the American and Canadian health care systems focusing on differences in funding, management, and operation. This is shown through a comparison of American and Canadian patients with similar medical problems. (60 minute videocassette)

Filmaker's Library. <u>What's ailing medicine</u>? New York: Author. This video addresses the issues of providing health care for the 37 million Americans who do not have insurance, providing better health care for those whose insurance is inadequate, and controlling the mounting costs of today's health care. Hillary Rodham Clinton and Senator Robert Dole give their views on the issue. (58 minute videocassette)

National Health Program Coalition. <u>Canada's national health program: A model for the United States</u>? Berkeley, CA: Author. [1300 Shattuck Ave. Suite A, Berkeley, CA 94709]. On this videocassette Canadians, physicians, economists, consumers and others, tell Americans about their National Health Program. They discuss its universal coverage, financing, choice of doctor and hospital, advanced technology, and satisfaction with their system. Filmed in Vancouver, Canada. (27 minute videocassette)

NBC News. <u>The Brokaw report. America's health care: going broke in style</u>. New York: Author. Factors which contribute to the health care crisis in the United States are examined. Included are: use of emergency rooms by the poor, insurance, refusal to allow hospitals to combine services, and unnecessary procedures to guard against malpractice suits. A group of health care experts discuss issues at the end. (48 minute videocassette)

UNIT IV

ENVIRONMENTAL HEALTH AND SAFETY

CHAPTER 15

Environmental Concerns: Wastes and Pollution

CHAPTER SYNOPSIS

In this chapter, the first of two on environmental issues in community health, we introduce the concept of the environment as a system. We then review the various types of wastes and pollution produced in our communities. For each type of waste or pollutant, we outline the sources and summarize present and future solutions for reduction and control. In the next chapter we address specific health risks that can result from mismanaging our environment.

CHAPTER OUTLINE

I.   Introduction

    A.   As human beings, we are part of the environment.

    B.   The way in which we interact with our environment influences the quality of our lives.

II. The Environmental System: The environmental system can be considered to have four major components.

    A.   Life support systems include all aspects of the environment that provide a basis for life.

        1.   Energy

        2.   Geographical systems

        3.   The biological system

        4.   Items built by humans

        5.   Social interaction among humans

    B.   Human activities include all human activities from growing of food to building of homes; and from recreating to making war.

    C.   Residues and wastes are the by-products of human activities including human wastes, energy production wastes, transportation wastes, etc.

        1.   Human body wastes: urine and feces

        2.   Excess materials and foods: trash and garbage

3. Vegetation wastes: grass clippings and tree branches

4. Construction and manufacturing wastes: scrap wood, metal and stone, contaminated water, solvents, and excess heat and noise.

5. Transportation wastes: carbon monoxide, nitrous oxides, hydrocarbons, other gaseous pollutants and used motor oil

6. Energy production wastes: mining wastes, electrical power (combustion of coal), nuclear power (radioactive) wastes and weapons production (radioactive) wastes

D. Environmental hazards are products or occurrences that are destructive to the environment.

1. Site and location hazards

2. Biological hazards

3. Chemical hazards

4. Physical hazards

5. Physiological hazards

6. Sociological hazards

III. Wastes and Pollution

A. Wastes and residues are being generated faster than they are being removed.

B. Four factors have contributed to this phenomenon.

1. Urbanization

2. Industrialization

3. Population growth

4. Production of disposable containers and products

IV. Solid wastes include garbage, trash, yard waste, wood, metal, stone and glass scrapes from domestic or industrial sources.

A. Sources of solid waste

1. Agriculture

2. Mining

3. Industry

4. Municipal sources

B. Solid waste management

1. Collection is the gathering and transporting of solid wastes from the point of origin to the point of disposal.

2. Disposal is the final disposition of solid wastes in such a way as to prevent them from harming the environment or human health.

   a. Sanitary landfills are sites or locations judged suitable for the in-ground disposal of solid wastes.

   b. Incineration is the burning or combustion of solid wastes.

3. Recycling (resource recovery) is the collection and reprocessing of a solid waste "resource" so it can be reused.

   a. Composting of garbage and yard wastes

   b. Recycling of soft drink cans and bottles

4. Source reduction is the reduction in, or elimination of use of materials that could become solid waste.

V. Hazardous Wastes are those that are dangerous to human health or to the environment.

A. Hazardous wastes are solid wastes that can:

1. Cause or significantly contribute to an increase in mortality or an increase in serious irreversible, or incapacitating, reversible illness.

2. Pose a substantial present or potential hazard to human health or the environment when improperly treated, stored, transported, or disposed of, or otherwise managed.

B. Hazardous waste management

1. Secured landfills are the least expensive method of hazardous waste disposal when they are:

   a. Carefully designed and located

   b. Monitored for leakage

2. Deep well injection is the pumping of liquid hazardous waste into wells below the aquifer.

3. Incineration of hazardous waste is the controlled combustion of hazardous waste.

4. Hazardous waste recycling is the process of reusing hazardous waste to produce a usable product, a process sometimes accomplished through "waste exchanges" in Europe.

5. Neutralization of hazardous waste is the process of detoxifying the waste so it is less toxic, corrosive, or otherwise hazardous.

6. Source reduction is the alteration of manufacturing processes to reduce or eliminate the generation of hazardous waste.

C. Hazardous waste cleanup

    1. Since the disposal of hazardous waste was unregulated before 1976, there exist many hazardous waste sites around the United States.

    2. The "Superfund" Law (CERCLA) was passed in 1980 and amended in 1986 to clean up such sites.

VI. Air pollution is the contamination of the air by substances in amounts great enough to interfere with comfort, safety and health.

A. Air pollution can arise from both natural and human sources.

B. Air pollution can occur indoors as well as outdoors.

C. Sources of outdoor air pollution include:

    1. Transportation

    2. Electric

    3. Power generation

    4. Industry

D. The Pollutant Standard Index is a scale that relates pollution concentrations to health effects.

E. Special concerns with outdoor air include: Acid rain, destruction of the ozone layer, global warming and photochemical smog.

    1. Acid rain refers to the deposition on the earth surface of sulfuric and nitrous acids removed from the atmosphere during the formation of rain droplets.

        a. Acid rain can damage vegetation and human structures.

        b. Acid rain often falls on areas distant to the pollution source.

    2. The ozone layer surrounds the earth and filters out a significant portion of the sun's ultraviolet radiation.

        a. Chlorofluorocarbons, a group of industrial chemicals, is believed to be partly responsible for depleting the ozone layer.

        b. Industrialized countries have agreed to stop or reduce the use of CFCs.

    3. Global warming is the gradual increase in the earth's temperature.

        a. There is still controversy among scientists as to whether global warming is actually occurring.

        b. It may be that the building up of greenhouse gases will trap heat radiated by the earth's surface and cause global warming.

    4. Photochemical smog is a secondary air pollutant created when primary pollutants react with sunlight and atmospheric oxygen.

    a.   Denver, Los Angeles, Phoenix and Salt Lake City all experience photochemical smog.

    b.   Thermal inversions, the trapping of cooler air under warmer air, worsen the effects of photochemical smog.

D. Protection of outdoor air through regulation dates to 1815 in Pittsburgh, Pennsylvania.

    1.   Air quality in the U.S. deteriorated until the Clean Air Act was passed in 1963.

    2.   The first Earth Day was celebrated in 1970, the same year that the Environmental Protection Agency was established and important amendments to the Clean Air Act were passed.

E. Indoor air

    1.   As outdoor air has become cleaner, there has been more concern about the quality of indoor air.

    2.   Indoor air pollutants are gases or particulate matter inside buildings that interfere with human comfort, safety and health.

        a.   Asbestos

        b.   Aeroallergens

        c.   Combustion by-products

        d.   Formaldehyde

        e.   Radon

        f.   Environmental tobacco smoke

        g.   Volatile organic compounds

    3.   Protection of indoor air quality can be achieved by changes in policy and/or individual behavior.

        a.   Policy to regulate indoor air quality is generally aimed at smoking.

        b.   Individual behavioral changes represent an important way to improve indoor air quality.

VII. Water and Its Pollution

A. Sources of water

    1.   Surface water includes water from lakes, reservoirs, rivers and streams.

    2.   Ground water lies in aquifers many feet below the earth's surface.

    3.   Salt water must be desalinized before use.

B. Treatment of water for domestic use

1. Municipal water treatment plants provide water that is chemically and biologically safe for human consumption.

2. Treatment of surface water includes several cleaning steps and then disinfection.

C. Water pollution can be point source and non-point source pollution.

1. Point source pollution occurs at a single point, for example and industrial plant.

2. Non-point source pollution is all other pollution in water.

D. Water pollutants can be biological, toxic or of various other types.

1. Biological pollutants are living agents

a. Viruses, bacterial and other parasites

b. Overgrowth of plant life in water source

2. Toxic pollutants

a. Inorganic chemicals such as lead, copper, etc.

b. Radioactive pollution

c. Synthetic organic compounds such as pesticides

3. Miscellaneous pollutants

a. Oil such as oil tanker spills

b. Thermal pollution (heated water)

E. Water Related Issues

1. Water quantity

a. Overall there is ample freshwater in America.

b. Certain areas have experienced droughts resulting in water shortages.

2. Water quality in the United States is threatened by four conditions

a. Population growth

b. Growth of the chemical industry

c. Environmental mismanagement, including irresponsible waste disposal

d. Reckless land use practices

F. Strategies to insure safe water -date to John Snow and the cholera epidemic in London in 1849.

1. Water quality legislation

    a. Federal Water Pollution Control Act Amendments (1972) was the first comprehensive federal water quality law.

    b. Clean Water Act (1977) required that all rivers in America be swimmable and fishable and the discharge of pollutants into United States water be zero.

    c. Safe Drinking Water Act (1974) instructed the EPA to set maximum contaminant levels for specific pollutants in drinking water.

2. Waste water treatment is the removal of organic wastes from waste water or their conversion to inorganic wastes so that they do not unduly enrich receiving waters.

    a. <u>Primary treatment</u> is the separation of liquids and solids in waste water.

        i. Solid waste is sludge and passes to sludge digestion

        ii. Liquid (aqueous) waste enters secondary treatment

    b. <u>Secondary treatment</u> involves the addition of bacteria (activated sludge), aeration, trickling filters, settling ponds.

    c. <u>Tertiary treatment</u> (advanced sewage treatment) involves sand and charcoal filters.

    d. <u>Septic systems</u> are waste water treatment systems for those who live in unsewered areas.

3. Conservation of water

    a. On average, each American generates about 100 gallons of waste water each day.

    b. Water conservation could reduce the amount substantially.

VIII. Radiation

  A. Radiation is the energy released when an atom is split.

    1. Radiation travels in waves or particles.

    2. Uncontrolled radiation can be hazardous to human health.

  B. Sources of radiation can be natural or human-made.

    1. Naturally occurring radiation comes from three sources.

        a. The sun and outer space

        b. The earth and its minerals

        c. Inside the body from ingestion

    2. Human-made radiation

        a. X-rays

      b.   Nuclear medicine

      c.   Nuclear weapons

  C. The danger of radiation

     1.   Excess radiation can damage cells and tissues.

     2.   Radiation doses are measured in REMS (Roentgen equivalent man).

  D. Policy related to nuclear waste disposal

     1.   United States Department of Energy is responsible for the safe disposal of nuclear waste.

     2.   Nuclear waste disposal is a highly controversial issue.

IX. Noise Pollution can be defined as excess noise.

  A. What is noise and how is it measured?

     1.   Noise is the result of energy conversion to vibrations that are detected by instruments and our ears.

     2.   Noise has various qualities such as frequency and amplitude.

  B. Approaches to noise abatement

     1.   Policy

        a.   Most policies that deal with noise are local policies.

        b.   Noise Control Act of 1972 was the first federal law on noise control and dealt with consumer products only.

     2.   Educational programs aimed at reducing noise are unproven in their effectiveness.

     3.   Environmental modifications offer solutions for reducing noise in some situations.

TEACHING IDEAS

Writing Assignment. At the beginning of this chapter before you present any of the information from the text, ask your students to write on a piece of paper the description of any situations where the environment in their hometown was being or had been polluted. Ask them to describe the situation, how they became aware of it, and what was done to abate the situation. Ask if anyone in the class would be willing to share his/her experience. Let several respond. This type of discussion provides many examples to use when discussing Purdon's description of the environmental system.

Field Trip. The content of this chapter provides a lot of opportunity for field trips. Suggested sites include but are not limited to: a sanitary or secured landfill, a water treatment plant, and a hazardous waste clean-up site.

ANNOTATED REFERENCES

Baechler, M. et at. (1991). <u>Sick building syndrome: Sources, health effects, mitigation</u> <u>(Pollution technology review no. 205)</u>. Park Ridge, NJ: Noyes Data Corp. This text examines the sources of indoor air pollution, ventilation, and possible solutions to the problem. It also includes information on specific hazardous contaminants that have been found in the indoor air in public buildings.

Chiras, D. (1994). <u>Environmental science: Action for a sustainable future</u> (4th ed.). Redwood City, CA: Benjamin/Cummings Publishing Co., Inc. This book investigates the causes of environmental problems concerning population, resources, and pollution issues. The focus is on positive action for dealing with environmental concerns through an understanding of environmental issues.

Cranor, C. (1993). <u>Regulating toxic substances: A philosophy of science and the law</u>. New York: Oxford University Press. The author examines the differences between scientific and legal standards concerning the issues connected with toxic substances. He also discusses the problems in trying to regulate human exposure to these substances.

Fay, F. (Ed.). (1991). <u>Noise & health</u>. New York: New York Academy of Medicine. This text begins with an overview and a definition of noise. Contributing authors then discuss physiological, psychological, and sociological effects of noise on humans. The last several chapters focus on community responses to noise, strategies for controlling noise, legislation, and public awareness and education concerning the ill effects of noise.

Morgan, M. (1993). <u>Environmental health</u>. Madison, WI: Brown & Benchmark. This comprehensive text gives an overview of a wide range of environmental health issues. Topics include: world population, fundamentals of environmental health, disease, water supplies and treatment, solid and hazardous waste management, vector control, radiological health, food quality control, air quality, environmental laws, and occupational health.

ANNOTATED AUDIOVISUALS

Chedd-Angier Production Company. <u>Toxic trials</u>. Northbrook, IL: Coronet Film & Video. This video studies the origin of hazardous waste in Woburn, Massachusetts, and attempts to determine the extent of contamination. It also looks at possible health effects, particularly, leukemia. (60 minute videocassette)

Churchill Films. <u>Garbage, the movie: An environmental crisis</u>. Los Angeles, CA: Author. This video examines the solid waste problem in our environment and offers several solutions. (25 minute videocassette)

Earthtalk. <u>Don't give me that trash!</u> Bozeman, MT: Author. This program uses Montana as an example for ways of recycling in a community. It also shows how recycled products can be made into new products, saving valuable resources.

Films for the Humanities & Sciences. <u>Saving the Water</u>. Princeton, NJ: Author. [P. O. Box 2053, Princeton, NJ 08543-2053]. Using issues relating to the Rhine River and the Colorado River, this program illustrates the delicate balance between the need and availability of water. It addresses the problems of global warming and political conflicts as they relate to water supply. (15 minute videocassette)

Films for the Humanities & Sciences. <u>Saving the Planet</u>. Princeton, NJ: Author. [P. O. Box 2053, Princeton, NJ 08543-2053]. This program looks at three case studies relating to improving the environment. The first is an energy conservation program developed by an Iowa community; the second is an example of technology serving the environment developed by Volvo; and the last is a tree planting endeavor in Kenya to counterbalance deforestation. (15 minute videocassette)

CHAPTER 16

The Impact of Environment on Human Health

CHAPTER SYNOPSIS

In the previous chapter, Chapter 15, we described the environment as a system and presented information about various types of wastes and pollutants. In this chapter, we explain how these wastes and pollutants affect human health. These hazards are divided into six groups and each group is discussed in turn. For each group of hazards, organized community health efforts to control or reduce the health risks are described.

CHAPTER OUTLINE

I.   Introduction

    A.   The environment is all that affects an organism during its lifetime.

    B.   Environmental health refers to characteristics of the environment that affect human health.

    C.   These may be biological, chemical, physical, psychological, sociological or site and location hazards.

II. Biological hazards are living organisms that are harmful to humans.

    A.   Water-borne diseases are diseases that are transmitted in drinking water.

        1.   Examples are poliovirus, hepatitis A virus, Shigella, Cholera, amoebic dysentery, Giardia and Crytosporidium.

        2.   These disease organisms are shed into the water in feces.

        3.   Our municipal water treatment facilities usually are able to purify water by removing these agents or disinfecting the water.

        4.   Occasional outbreaks of water-borne diseases continue to occur.

        5.   Hard pesticides such as the now banned DDT remained in the environment for months or years.

        6.   Soft pesticides, the ones most commonly used today, break down in hours or days.

    B.   Food-borne diseases are diseases transmitted in or on food.

1. Examples of food-borne agents are <u>Salmonella</u>, <u>Clostridium botulinum</u>, <u>Staphylococcus aureus</u>, <u>Clostridium perfingens</u> and <u>Shigella</u>.

2. To protect against food-borne diseases, sanitarians from local health departments routinely inspect food service establishments (restaurants), and retail food outlets (supermarkets) to verify that food is being stored and handled properly.

III. Chemical hazards result from the presence of concentrations of substances or materials that are hazardous to health. Examples are pesticides, lead and tobacco smoke.

A. Pesticides are chemicals that have been manufactured for the purpose of reducing populations of undesirable organisms.

1. Examples of categories of pesticides are herbicides and insecticides.

2. Most pesticides kill non-target organisms as well as the target or pest species.

3. The wise use of pesticides can protect human health and agricultural crops.

4. Misuse of pesticides can result in illness and death.

B. Environmental tobacco smoke is an environmental hazard produced by the 45.8 million Americans that smoke.

1. Diseases associated with ETS include lung cancer and perhaps heart disease.

2. ETS contains 4,000 substances.

3. The EPA has classified ETS as a Class A carcinogen.

4. Smoking has been increasingly restricted from public buildings and from many private worksites.

5. Regulation of smoking seems to be the best approach to controlling this pollutant.

C. Lead is a naturally occurring element that is used in the manufacturing of many industrial and domestic products.

1. Health problems associated with the over exposure to lead are anemia, birth defects, bone damage, neurological damage, kidney damage and others.

2. Exposure is by ingestion and inhalation.

3. Children are particularly at risk from eating peeling lead paint.

4. Other sources include the lead in gasoline, water pipes and drinking water tainted by lead leached from landfills.

5. Occupational exposure is another source of lead.

6. Solutions for the prevention of lead poisoning include education, regulation and prudent behavior.

IV. Physical hazards include airborne particles, humidity, equipment design and radiation.

A. Ultraviolet radiation reaches humans as short wave length energy that can damage cells by ionization.

    1. One result of over exposure to UV radiation is skin cancer.

    2. People should reduce their exposure to UV radiation.

        a. Stay inside

        b. Wear protective clothes or sunscreen

B. Radon contamination results from over exposure to radon gas.

    1. Radon gas arises naturally from the earth and sometimes occurs at dangerous levels in buildings and homes.

    2. Breathing in radon gas can cause lung cancer.

    3. Homes can be tested for the presence of radon gas for $20.

V. Psychological hazards are environmental factors that produce psychological changes expressed as stress, depression, hysteria and hypochondriasis. This topic is more extensively covered in Chapter 11.

VI. Sociological hazards are those that result from living in a society where one experiences noise, lack of privacy and overcrowding.

A. Population growth may be a sociological hazard.

    1   Principles

        a. Growth of living populations can be expressed as an S curve with a lag phase, log phase and equilibrium phase.

        b. When environmental resources can support no further growth, the population has reached the equilibrium phase and the environment is said to be at its carrying capacity.

    2. Facts

        a. The human population is now in log-phase (exponential) growth.

        b. Growth rates are faster for populations of underdeveloped nations.

        c. Exponential growth cannot be maintained indefinitely.

    3. Issues

        a. Exponential growth means community health problems will increase.

        b. It also means that most environmental problems will worsen.

    4. Solutions

        a. Population growth will eventually be limited either by human initiative or by nature.

      b.   Human initiatives aimed at curbing population growth would be more humane than nature's.

VII. Site and Location Hazards and Human Health

    A.   Natural disasters are geographical and meteorological events of such magnitude and proximity to communities that they produce significant damage and injuries.

        1.   Examples are cyclones, earthquakes, floods, hurricanes, tornadoes, typhoons and volcanic eruptions.

        2.   The magnitude of devastation of these events can sometimes be great.

        3.   Biological, psychological and sociological hazards may increase following a natural disaster.

        4.   Federal, state and local agencies often provide help to clean up the damage and prevent a biological, psychological or sociological disaster from following a physical one.

TEACHING IDEAS

Guest Speaker. After you have covered the material presented in this chapter, invite a representative from the American Red Cross (ARC) Disaster Services Committee to discuss the procedures the ARC goes through when they are asked to respond to a site and location hazard. Have the speaker start with how the ARC knows when to respond to a hazard through the last step of discontinuing service. As with all guest speakers, you may want to have your students write questions for which they would like the speaker to respond. This should be done the class session before the scheduled date of the speaker in order to group like questions.

Role Play Situation. Create a skit dealing with a controversial environmental health issue such as smoking in public places, birth control in third world countries, or the building of a nuclear power plant. Have several of your students put on the skit, then let the rest of the class respond to it by writing a one paragraph solution to the problem. Ask several students to read their response, then open it up to a class discussion.

ANNOTATED REFERENCES

Blumenthal, D. & Ruttenber, J. (1994). Introduction to environmental health (2nd ed.). New York: Springer Publishing Co. This is a valuable resource for students in almost all health-related fields. It provides an overview of environmental health and contains information on health promotion.

Hall, R. (1990). Health and the global environment. Colchester, VT: Basil Blackwell, Inc. This text is divided into two sections. The first is, "Health Care and Attitudes Toward the Environment," focusing on the ideas that if the quality of the environment were improved, many health problems would be avoided. The second section, "Environment and the Preventive Approach," examines environmental issues from a worldwide perspective.

Lappe, M. (1991). Chemical deception: The toxic threat to health and the environment. San Francisco, CA: Sierra Club Books. The author examines toxic contaminants of the environment and their effects on humans. He discusses ten "myths" about chemicals that are hazardous to everyone. He also suggests better methods to study and evaluate the problem, and advocates basic guidelines and rules for protecting the environment and those who live in it.

Moeller, D. (1992). <u>Environmental health: A guide for public health professionals.</u> Cambridge, MA: Harvard University Press. The author examines environmental health concerns by discussing personal, indoor, outdoor, and worldwide environments. He covers a broad range of topics such as: indoor and outdoor air, water and sewage, foodborne disease, solid waste, rodents and insects, injuries, radiation, energy sources, and man-made disasters.

Upton, A. & Graber, E. (1993). <u>Staying healthy in a risky environment.</u> Tacoma, WA: Apple A Day Books. This text, from the New York University Med Center, discusses how to identify, prevent, or minimize environmental risks that affect the health of individuals.

ANNOTATED AUDIOVISUALS

Commonweal Productions. <u>Air pollution.</u> Cambridge, MA: Author. This video examines the sources of air pollution and considers its impact on our health. It also looks at state and federal regulatory programs and makes predictions for improved air quality in the future.

Films for the Humanities & Sciences. <u>Saving the Atmosphere.</u> Princeton, NJ: Author. [P. O. Box 2053, Princeton, NJ 08543-2053]. This program focuses on smog in the city of Los Angeles; the causes and the effects on human beings. It also examines other issues such as the greenhouse effect and massive coastal flooding. (15 minute videocassette)

Films for the Humanities & Sciences. <u>Saving the Land.</u> Princeton, NJ: Author. [P. O. Box 2053, Princeton, NJ 08543-2053]. This video examines waste disposal; where it goes, how it affects the environment, and how recycling can help. It also discusses the use of pesticides and their effects on humans and animals. Also appropriate for Chapter 15. (15 minute videocassette)

Films for the Humanities & Sciences. <u>Smokers are Hazardous.</u> Princeton, NJ: Author. [P. O. Box 2053, Princeton, NJ 08543-2053]. This BBC Horizon program looks at the risks of secondary smoke and smoking related illnesses among non smokers. It provides an insight into those who make money from promoting tobacco, and smokers themselves who endanger themselves and others by refusing to give up smoking. (50 minute videocassette)

Public Interest Video Network. <u>Your water, your life.</u> Northbrook, IL: Film Ideas. This production studies the problem of our nation's contaminated ground water supply and explains how individuals are dealing with the problem. (28 minute 30 second videocassette)

CHAPTER 17

Injuries as a Community Health Problem

CHAPTER SYNOPSIS

In this chapter we define and examine the scope of both unintentional injuries and intentional injuries as community health problems. Not only are these among the leading causes of death, but are also leading causes of years of potential life lost, of lost productivity and of disability. We also discuss approaches to reducing the number and seriousness of unintentional and intentional injuries.

CHAPTER OUTLINE

I. Introduction

    A. Definitions

        1. Injury is physical harm or damage resulting from an acute exchange of energy that exceeds the body's tolerance.

        2. Unintentional injuries are those judged to have occurred without anyone intending harm to be done.

        3. Intentional injuries are injuries that have been purposefully inflicted whether by oneself or another.

    B. Cost of injuries to society

        1. Each year more than 150,000 people die from fatal injuries.

        2. This includes approximately 45,000 motor vehicle deaths, 55,000 other unintentional injury deaths and 50,000 intentional injury deaths.

        3. There are 57 million Americans injured each year because of foregone productivity, and costs of hospitalization and rehabilitation.

        4. Disabling injuries cost this country billions of dollars each year because of foregone productivity, and costs of hospitalization and rehabilitation.

        5. Injuries are the fourth leading cause of death in the U.S. but the first leading cause of lost productivity.

II. Unintentional Injuries

A. Types of unintentional injuries

   1. Unintentional injuries, by themselves, are the fourth leading cause of death in the United States.

   2. In 1991, fatal and nonfatal unintentional injuries cost Americans approximately $177 billion.

   3. Motor vehicle crashes

      a. The leading cause of unintentional injury deaths is motor vehicle crashes.

      b. In 1990, there were 44,531 fatalities, 5.4 million non-fatal injuries and 28 million damaged vehicles.

   4. Other types of unintentional injuries

      a. Examples of other causes of unintentional injuries are falls, fires, drownings, suffocation and the discharge of firearms.

      b. Other causes include transport deaths such as those that occur during air, water, or rail travel, or on street cars and bicycles.

B. The epidemiology of unintentional injuries can be examined by person, place and time.

   1. Person

      a. Age - unintentional injuries are the leading cause of death in the 1-44 year age group.

      b. Sex - males are twice as likely to suffer a fatal unintentional injury as females.

      c. Race - black males have more unintentional injury deaths than white males. Native American males have the highest unintentional injury fatality rate of any group.

   2. Place

      a. Home - more unintentional injuries occur in the home than in any other place.

      b. Residential institutions - following the home, the next highest rate of unintentional injuries occurs in residential institutions.

      c. Workplace - Workplace ranks third as a place for unintentional injuries.

      d. Highway - more unintentional injury fatalities occur on the highways than anywhere else.

   3. Time -unintentional injury rates vary with season.

      a. More drownings occur in the summer months

      b. More deaths from fires occur in the winter months

    c.   More motor vehicle deaths occur at night

    4.   Alcohol and other drugs as risk factors

        a.   Alcohol may be the single most important factor associated with both intentional and unintentional injuries.

        b.   About half of fatal motor vehicle crashes involved alcohol.

        c.   Alcohol is involved in nearly half of adult drownings.

        d.   In one study, more than half of adult cyclists with brain injuries were legally intoxicated at the time of their injury.

C.   Prevention through epidemiology

    1.   Early contributors to injury prevention and control

        a.   Hugh De Haven designed vehicle interiors for greater safety.

        b.   John E. Gordon proposed using the methods of epidemiology to study the causes of injuries.

        c.   William Haddon, Jr. insisted that research on accident prevention be developed into public policy.

    2.   A model for unintentional injuries incorporates energy as the agent in the standard public health model of agent, host and environment.

    3.   Prevention and control tactics based upon the public health model stress interrupting transmission of damaging energy to the host.

        a.   Prevent accumulation of energy

        b.   Prevent the inappropriate release of energy

        c.   Place a barrier between humans and energy

        d.   Completely exclude humans from proximity to energy source

    4.   Other tactics

        a.   Strengthen educational programs

        b.   Strengthen EMS response capabilities

        c.   Strengthen ordinances against dangerous behaviors

D.   Community based approaches to the prevention of unintentional injuries.

    1.   Education is the process of changing people's health directed behavior to reduce unintentional injuries.

    2.   Regulation is the enactment and enforcement of laws to control conduct to reduce unintentional injuries.

3. Automatic protection is the technique of designing a product or the environment to reduce unintentional injuries.

4. Litigation is the process of seeking justice for injury through the courts.

III. Intentional Injuries are the Outcome of Self-Directed or Interpersonal Violence

    A. Scope of the problem

        1. Approximately 50,000 people die each year from intentional injuries.

        2. About 2.2 million receive nonfatal injuries as a result of interpersonal violence.

    B. Types of intentional injuries

        1. Assaults

        2. Family Violence

        3. Rape

        4. Robbery

        5. Suicide

        6. Homicide

    C. Rates of violent acts in the United States based on 1991 records

        1. There were 35 million violent crimes committed or attempted.

        2. Homicide was the 9th leading cause of death.

        3. Suicide was the 8th leading cause of death.

        4. Suicides accounted for one-fifth of all injury deaths.

    D. Epidemiology of intentional injuries

        1. Interpersonal violence disproportionately affects those who are jobless, hopeless, poor and have low self-esteem.

        2. More violent acts are committed by males.

        3. Perpetrators of violent acts are more likely to have been abused as children.

        4. Rates of homicide, assault, and rape are highest among minorities.

            a. A black American male in 1989 had a 1 in 27 chance of becoming a murder victim vs. 1 in 205 for a white male.

            b. Many victims are women who are battered.

            c. Only half of all rape victims report the crime.

        5. Suicide and attempted suicide

     a.   Nearly 30,000 suicides are reported each year.

     b.   Men are three and one-half times more likely to commit suicide.

     c.   Suicide rates among the young have tripled since 1950.

6.   Firearm injuries

     a.   Firearm injuries are the second leading cause of injury deaths after motor vehicle crashes.

     b.   Sixty percent of homicide and 55% of suicides involved a firearm.

     c.   Males 15-34 years of age are at highest risk for death by firearms.

C.   Violence in our society

1.   Individuals and violence

     a.   Many individuals lack the communication and problem solving skills to settle disagreements nonviolently.

     b.   Firearms are easy to obtain and deadly.

     c.   Some conflict resolution programs have been developed to teach communication skills.

2.   Family violence and abuse

     a.   One in six homicides is the result of family violence.

     b.   Survivors of family violence are at greater risk for becoming violent as adults.

     c.   <u>Child abuse</u> is the intentional inflicting of physical, emotional, verbal or sexual injury upon a child.

     d.   <u>Child neglect</u> is the failure to provide necessary subsistence for a child - - physical, emotional or educational.

     e.   <u>Spouse Abuse</u> can be physical, emotional or sexual.

         i.   There are 2-4 million spouses abused each year.

         ii.   More than 1 million women seek medical attention for injuries received from domestic violence each year.

     f.   <u>A model for abuse</u> based upon the (triangular) public health model includes abuser, abused and crisis.

         i.   A crisis can arise from a loss of a job, divorce or child misbehavior.

         ii.   Alcohol and other drug use are conditions that increase the risk that violence will occur.

3.   Gangs and violence

      a.   Youth gangs have been around a long time.

      b.   Violence has increased recently because of the availability of drugs, the money to be made selling drugs, and easy access to firearms.

      c.   Gang related homicides increased from 271 in 1979 to 771 in 1991.

      d.   There are 1,000 nonfatal injuries for each fatality.

      e.   Gangs and gang related violence place enormous demand on law enforcement agencies.

      f.   Gangs deface property which is costly to repair.

      g.   Community response should be multifaceted and include: law enforcement, education, diversion activities, and social services support.

D.   Approaches to prevention of intentional injuries

    1.   Education

      a.   Parenting skills for adults

      b.   Nonviolent problem solving skills for youth

      c.   Self-esteem raising programs for youths and adults

    2.   Opportunities for employment and recreation

      a.   Jobs programs

      b.   Recreation programs

    3.   Regulation and enforcement

      a.   The "Brady Bill" regulates hand gun purchases

      b.   Electronic detection of weapons

      c.   Other types of regulation

    4.   Counseling and treatment represent secondary and tertiary prevention

E.   A comprehensive approach includes improved surveillance and training, community empowerment and evaluation of existing programs.

    1.   Reduction in injuries resulting from firearm violence

      a.   Education and behavioral changes

      b.   Technological and environmental efforts

      c.   Enhanced enforcement of existing laws

      d.   New legislation and regulation

2. Reduction in use of alcohol and other drugs

    a. Decrease chronic use by high risk individuals -treatment

    b. Prevent first use by high risk individuals

    c. Review current drug laws

3. Improvement of childhood experiences

    a. Home visitation programs

    b. Educational intervention

    c. Crisis intervention programs

4. Prevention and management of mental disorders.

    a. Better treatment

    b. Expand training for professionals who are gatekeepers for treatment services

    c. Increase funding for out patient treatment of patients with mental disorders

TEACHING IDEAS

Newspaper Clippings. Prior to presenting the content of this chapter, scan your local newspaper looking for articles that are related to unintentional or intentional injuries. Cut the articles out of the paper and have them made into overhead transparencies. Show them to the students at the beginning of class. Talk about each of the articles and ask the students if such injuries could be prevented. Ask them to defend their answer. Then ask what the community could do to prevent such injuries.

Writing Assignment. This activity could be conducted at the beginning or end of the lesson that covers the content in this chapter. Have the students respond in writing to the following stem "Drunk driving could be prevented if..." Have several students share their response with the rest of the class and have the other students either agree or disagree with the rationale. If the activity is conducted at the beginning of the class it can be used at a springboard for the rest of the class time. If it is used at the end of the class, students can be asked to defend their response based on the information presented in text.

ANNOTATED REFERENCES

Cervantes, R. (Ed.). (1992). Substance abuse and gang violence. Newbury Park, CA: SAGE Publications. This text is a good resource for students in social work, psychology, psychiatry, and public health. It provides information for the development of community-based prevention and intervention programs.

Kilgore, N. (1993). Every 18 seconds: A journey through domestic violence. Volcano, CA: Volcano Press, Inc. This book provides information for an understanding of domestic violence. It is especially helpful for women who have been abused.

Martin, D. (1981). Battered wives. Volcano, CA: Volcano Press, Inc. This book addresses the problem of wife abuse and provides critical summaries of the legal and political status of battered wives.

Sonkin, D. & Durphy, M. (1989). <u>Learning to live without violence</u>. Volcano, CA: Volcano Press, Inc. This book suggests ways to control anger, discusses drug and alcohol use, and explains ways to deal with feelings of alienation and jealousy.

Starr, R. & Wolfe, D. (Eds.). (1991). <u>The effects of child abuse and neglect</u>: Issues in research. New York: Guilford Press. This book examines child abuse and its effects on individuals throughout their lives. Contents include an analysis of a longitudinal study, a study of measurement questions for parental personality characteristics, parent-child interactions, and the emotional status of abused children.

ANNOTATED AUDIOVISUALS

Filmakers. <u>Rape prevention: Trust your instincts</u>. Northbrook, IL: MTI Film & Video. This program offers a workshop for women showing them how to prevent sexual assault.

Films for the Humanities & Sciences. <u>Childhood sexual abuse</u>. Princeton, NJ: Author. [P.O. Box 2053, Princeton, NJ 08543-2053]. Through reports from psychiatrists, social workers, and law enforcement officials, this program looks at the child abuse pattern in families, signs of sexual abuse, reporting procedures, and prevention. (26 minute videocassette)

Films for the Humanities & Sciences. <u>Injury prevention</u>. Princeton, NJ: Author. [P.O. Box 2053, Princeton, NJ 08543-2053]. This video examines risk-taking behavior and the most common areas of danger. Avoiding injury through common sense is explored. (26 minute videocassette)

Films for the Humanities & Sciences. <u>No more secrets</u>. Princeton, NJ: Author. [P.O. Box 2053, Princeton, NJ 08543-2053]. This program examines long term effects of sexual abuse by focusing on particular children and adults who were abused. (24 minute videocassette)

Lifetime Productions. <u>Against her will: Rape on campus.</u> Coronet/MTI Film & Video. This video looks at case studies of acquaintance rape on campuses in the United States, and how these incidents can be prevented.

WETA- TV. <u>Drinking and driving: the toll, the tears.</u> Washington, DC: Author. This Phil Donahue program explores how a drunken driver changed people's lives. Individuals share their stories from a home, a prison, a church, a hospital, a prison, and a cemetery. (58 minute videocassette) This video is also appropriate for use in Chapter 12.

CHAPTER 18

Safety and Health in the Workplace

CHAPTER SYNOPSIS

In Chapter 17, we discussed unintentional and intentional injuries as public health problems. In this chapter, Chapter 18, we examine occupational injuries and disease. After reviewing the history and scope of the problem, we briefly outline legislative efforts aimed at protecting workers. We then discuss the epidemiology of occupational injuries and illnesses and review prevention and control efforts. Lastly, we outline resources (people and programs) for reducing the number and seriousness of workplace injuries and diseases.

CHAPTER OUTLINE

I. Introduction

   A. Scope of the problem

      1. The annual cost of occupational injuries, illnesses and deaths is estimated to be between $83 and $136 billion.

      2. The average cost per injury is $13,000.

      3. Between 7,000 and 11,000 workers die from work related injuries each year.

      4. Between 47,377 and 95,479 people die each year from occupational related disease.

   B. The importance of occupational safety and health to the community can be stated simply: The safety and health of the surrounding community is closely linked to safety and health in the workplace.

II. History of Occupational Safety and Health Problems

   A. Origins of the occupational safety and health movement

      1. The first writing on occupation safety and health of any type occurred in Europe in the 16th century.

      2. The first general work on the topic was Ramazzini's <u>Discourse on Diseases of Workers</u> which appeared in 1700.

   B. Occupational safety and health in the United States

1. The industrial revolution began in Britain and spread to the European continent and to the United States.

2. Power from burning coal resulted in larger factories with more workers.

3. As factory sizes increased, the number of injuries on the job also increased.

4. The first state legislation in the United States was a child labor law in Massachusetts.

5. Massachusetts also passed the first worker safety law in 1977.

6. The first Worker's Compensation law was passed in Maryland in 1902.

7. The first federal legislation was the Worker's Compensation law passed in 1908, a law which covered only certain federal employees.

C. Occupational Safety and Health Act of 1970 (OSHAct)

1. The purpose of the Occupational Safety and Health Act was to assure that employers in the private sector furnished each employee with employment and a worksite free from recognized hazards likely to cause death or serious physical harm.

2. The OSHAct required employers in the private sector to comply with standards promulgated and enforced by the Occupational Safety and Health Administration.

3. The OSHAct established both the Occupational Safety and Health Administration and the National Institute for Occupational Safety and Health (NIOSH).

4. NIOSH recommends occupational and safety and health standards.

III. Epidemiology of Occupational Injuries and Diseases

A. Occupational injuries are injuries that result from "a work accident or from exposure involving a single incident in the work environment."

1. Types of injuries

a. The leading cause of occupational injury deaths is motor vehicle crashes.

b. The leading type of non-fatal occupational injuries is back injuries.

c. These are also injuries to appendages and sense organs.

2. Injuries by age

a. Younger workers have more injuries than older workers.

b. Injury death rates are highest for workers 65 years and older.

c. Injuries in illegally employed children increased by 100% between 1983-1990.

3. Males sustain more injuries than females at every age.

4. Frequency of occupational injuries by income and race.

   a. Those in lower socioeconomic groups have higher occupational injury death rates.

   b. Occupation injury death rates are 12% higher in non-whites.

   c. Native Americans have high occupational injury death rates.

   d. Asians have low occupational injury death rates.

5. Frequency of occupational injuries by location.

   a. Occupational injury death rates per 100,000 workers are highest in mountain states and Alaska.

   b. Death rates from farm machinery injuries are highest in the north central states.

6. Distribution of occupational injuries by time.

   a. Overall injury rates per 100,000 workers have declined during this century, while production has increased.

   b. Injuries from work out of doors are highest in the summer.

7. Frequency of occupational injuries by type of job.

   a. Fatality rates are highest for mining, construction, transportation and agriculture.

   b. The most dangerous blue collar jobs are timber cutters/loggers; the most dangerous white collar job is that of an airplane pilot.

   c. Farming is also a hazardous occupation.

      i. There are still many tractors in use that are not equipped with rollover protection structures (ROPS).

      ii. Another group of agricultural workers at risk are migrant workers and their families. Working conditions for migrant workers are hazardous and living conditions are often unsanitary.

B. Controlling injuries in the workplace: The following working principles are in descending order of effectiveness.

   1. Modify the job to make it safer.

   2. Change the work environment to make it less hazardous.

   3. Redesign the machinery to make it safer.

   4. Improve the selection, training and education of the workers.

IV. Occupational Diseases

   A. More than 300,000 cases of occupational diseases were reported in 1990.

B. Leading types were repetitive trauma, skin disorders, and respiratory illnesses.

C. Types of diseases

    1. <u>Chronic musculoskeletal conditions</u> are the leading cause of disability in the workplace. Injury arises from continued trauma resulting inflamed, irritated or strained muscles, joints, tendons.

    2. <u>Dermatological conditions</u>

        a. Skin diseases are one of the 10 leading causes of workplace morbidity and disability.

        b. Examples are contact dermatitis, skin cancer and infections.

        c. Many toxic chemicals enter the body through the skin.

    3. <u>Occupational lung diseases</u> are caused by inhalation of toxic substances present in the workplace.

        a. Occupational lung diseases typically have a long latent period.

        b. Examples are asbestosis, byssinosis, silicosis and coal miner's pneumoconiosis.

    4. Other types of occupational diseases

        a. Neurological disorders

        b. Reproductive disorders

        c. Cardiovascular diseases

        d. Cancers

D. Controlling occupational diseases

    1. Vigilance of both employer and employee and assistance of the government is essential.

    2. There are specific activities that can be employed to control occupational disease.

    3. Occupational disease control programs require professionally trained personnel.

V. Resources for the Prevention of Occupational Injuries and Diseases

A. Occupational safety and health professionals include safety engineers, health physicists, industrial hygienists, occupational physicians, and occupational health nurses.

    1. Safety engineers and certified safety professionals design safety education programs and detect and correct or remove hazards in the workplace.

    2. Health physicists monitor radiation in the workplace and develop plans for decontamination and coping with radiation accidents.

3. Industrial hygienists are concerned with environmental factors in the workplace that might cause illness.

4. Occupational physicians are medical practitioners whose primary concern is preventive medicine in the workplace.

5. Occupational health nurses are registered nurses who practice in a workplace setting. Duties may range from first aid to health promotion and injury prevention.

B. Occupational safety and health programs have as their goal the hiring and maintaining of healthy workers.

1. Pre-placement examinations assure that applicants are physically matched for their jobs.

2. Health maintenance programs monitor employees for chronic health conditions and intervene to prevent a worsening of such problems.

3. Health promotion programs promote the health of employees to improve morale and productivity and to lower medical costs.

4. Safety programs are those portions of workplace health and safety programs aimed at reducing the number and seriousness of unintentional injuries on the job.

5. Employee assistance programs assist employees who have personal problems that interfere with job performance.

TEACHING IDEAS

Guest Speakers. Invite a "team" of safety employees in from a local industry. Try to get an administrator, a safety engineer, a health physicist, an industrial hygienist, and an occupational physician or nurse. Allow the speakers about half the time to talk about their jobs, responsibilities and the other half of the time to answer questions. In preparation for guest speakers to your classroom, have your students during the class period prior to the visit submit a question to you that they would like answered by the speakers. This will help to prepare the students for the speakers and personalize the experience for them. After the class, have the students write a short one paragraph summary on what the speakers presented.

Newspaper Clippings. Have your students read a newspaper to look for reports of occupational injuries, diseases, or deaths. Ask them to bring the articles to class to share with the others. This activity could be used at the beginning of the unit on occupational health as a springboard for the rest to the material presented in the chapter or at the end of the unit for analysis based upon new information learned.

ANNOTATED REFERENCES

Green, G. & Baker, F. (Eds.). (1991). Work, health, and productivity. New York: Oxford University Press. This book contains papers from the Johns Hopkins Conference on Work, Health, and Productivity. Contents include: a review of research, physical and chemical agents found in the workplace, genetic and environmental factors that contribute to biological susceptibility, changing physical and chemical natures of the workplace, psychosocial factors, cost of illness to an organization and health promotion.

National Safe Workplace Institute. (1992). <u>Basic information on workplace safety & health in the United States</u>. Chicago, IL: Author. This report provides a variety of information on workplace safety and health topics including: scope of the problem, demographics, enforcement and regulation, federal spending on job health, and workers' compensation. The three sections include statistical tables, a state-by-state analysis, and general information and concepts.

Robinson, J. (1991). <u>Toil and toxics: Workplace struggles and political strategies for occupational health</u>. Berkeley, CA: University of California Press. The author promotes the development of strategies to control workplace hazards. He describes four strategies designed to mitigate hazards in the workplace, including suggestions concerning workers's right to know, labor unions, and government regulation.

Wallerstein N. & Rubenstein, H. (1993). <u>Teaching about job hazards: A guide for workers and their health providers</u>. Washington, D.C.: APHA. This manual covers a variety of topics concerning occupational disease and injury. The authors believe that occupational disease and injury are almost totally preventable, and suggest guidelines on providing safety and health education to workers at risk.

Weeks, J., Levy, B., & Wagner, G. (Eds.). (1991). <u>Preventing occupational disease and injury</u>. Washington, D.C.: APHA. This handbook looks at occupational disease and injury from a public health point of view. Topics include: prevention and epidemiology, industrial hygiene, occupational medicine, injury control, regulatory resources, worker education and training.

ANNOTATED AUDIOVISUALS

American Lung Association. <u>Fight the flu and win</u>. Evans City, PA: Author. [P.O. Box 1036, Evans City, PA 16033]. This program focuses on health care workers and their susceptibility to contracting the flu. It explains what flu is and how a flu shot works, as well as when to get a flu shot. (10 minute videocassette)

American Lung Association. <u>Tuberculosis</u>. Evans City, PA: Author. This production discusses the detection of TB infection, transmission of TB, high risk individuals, and drug resistant TB. It also suggests practices for personal protection. (22 minute videocassette)

Filmakers Library. <u>Those who know don't tell: the ongoing battle for workers' health</u>. New York: Author. This production traces the history of workers' health risks from the early 1900s to the present, focusing on asbestos, mining, pesticides, and computer terminals. (29 minute videocassette)

Films for the Humanities & Sciences. <u>Industrial epidemics</u>. Princeton, NJ: Author. [P.O. Box 2053, Princeton, NJ 08543-2053]. This program looks at common work injuries, active rehabilitation and early intervention. It also suggests ways employers can minimize accidents and protect hearing and breathing of employees.

Women Make Movies, Inc. <u>Troubled harvest</u>. New York: Author. [225 Lafayette St., New York, NY 10012]. This video discusses the issues facing farmworkers today; child labor, pesticides, and immigration. The program looks at these problems from the farmworker woman's point of view. (30 minute videocassette)

TEST BANK

Chapter 1   Community Health -- Yesterday, Today, and Tomorrow

Multiple-Choice

Choose the one alternative that best completes the statement or answers the question.

1. The definition of health that states "health is a state of complete physical, mental, and social well-being and not merely the absence of disease and infirmity" was written in 1947 by
    A) Payne and Hahn.
    B) The World Health Organization.
    C) The Centers for Disease Control and Prevention.
    D) The Department of Health and Human Services.
    Answer: B

2. _____ is the sum of all official (governmental) efforts to promote, protect, and preserve the people's health.
    A) Community health
    B) Public health
    C) Personal health
    D) The concept of community
    Answer: B

3. A community is:
    A) a geographical area with specific boundaries
    B) a social unit that shares the same fate.
    C) defined by population size.
    Answer: B

4. With regard to the impact they have on the health of the community, what kind of factors do geography, the environment, community size, and industrial development represent?
    A) physical
    B) social
    C) cultural
    D) mental
    Answer: A

5. The percentage of people in the United States who smoke cigarettes today has_____ since 1960.
    A) increased
    B) decreased
    C) stayed about the same
    Answer: B

6. When the spread of a disease is slowed by a significant portion of the population being immunized against the disease it is called:
    A) mass immunization.
    B) active immunization.
    C) herd immunization.
    D) active immunity.
    Answer: C

7. The earliest written record concerning public health is the:
    A) Public Health Law of Rome.
    B) works of Shattuck.
    C) Greek Code of Health.
    D) Code of Hammurabi.
    Answer: D

8. Which of the periods in the history of community and public health is known as the "Spiritual Era of public health"?
    A) Ancient Societies
    B) Classical Cultures
    C) Middle Ages
    D) Renaissance and Exploration
    E) eighteenth, nineteenth and twentieth Centuries
    Answer: C

9. The deadliest of the epidemic diseases to date has been:
    A) syphilis.
    B) the plague.
    C) measles.
    D) A.I.D.S.
    E) influenza.
    Answer: B

10. The man credited with successfully demonstrating the process of vaccination as a protection against smallpox was:
    A) Dr. Edward Jenner.
    B) Louis Pasteur.
    C) Robert Koch.
    D) Dr. Thomas Wood.
    Answer: A

11. The modern era of public health began in:
    A) 1750.
    B) 1800.
    C) 1850.
    D) 1900.
    Answer: C

12. The germ theory of disease was proposed in 1862 by:
    A) Robert Koch.
    B) Edward Jenner.
    C) Louis Pasteur.
    D) Lamuel Shattuck.
    Answer: C

13. In his book The Jungle, Upton Sinclair wrote of the plight of the:
    A) workers in the steel mills of Pittsburgh.
    B) coal minors in West Virginia.
    C) immigrants working in the meat packing industry.
    D) cotton mill workers in South Carolina.
    Answer: C

14. The first national level volunteer health agency in the United States was the:
    A) National Association for the Study and Prevention of Tuberculosis.
    B) American Cancer Society.
    C) Pennsylvania Society for the Prevention of Tuberculosis.
    D) American Heart Association.
    Answer: A

15. The Public Health Service grew out of what earlier organization?
    A) The National Army-Navy Hospital
    B) The New England Health Service
    C) Marine Hospital Service
    D) Public Health U.S.A.
    Answer: C

16. Which one of the following did not occur in the 1930s?
    A) passage of the Social Security Act
    B) passage of the National Hospital Survey and Construction Act
    C) creation of President Franklin D. Roosevelt's New Deal
    D) formation of the National Cancer Institute
    Answer: B

17. A premature death is defined as any death prior to:
    A) age 65.
    B) retirement.
    C) the person's estimated life expectancy at birth.
    D) age 70.
    Answer: A

18. The only disease to be eradicated world wide was:
    A) mumps.
    B) tuberculosis.
    C) malaria.
    D) smallpox.
    Answer: D

19. Which of the following was (were) unknown only 20 years ago?
    A) Legionnaire's disease
    B) toxic shock syndrome
    C) Lyme disease
    D) AIDS
    E) all were unknown
    Answer: E

20. Which of the following is (are) projections for the United States in the year 2000?
    A) the population will reach nearly 270 million
    B) the percentage of white Americans will drop
    C) the percentage of women in the workplace will grow
    D) the median age of Americans will increase
    E) all are projections
    Answer: E

True-False

Write T if the statement is true and F if the statement is false.

1. By definition, communities do not necessarily require a political or governmental boundary.
   Answer: True

2. Some religious communities actively address moral and ethical issues like abortion, premaritial intercourse, and homosexuality.
   Answer: True

3. Alcohol consumption represents a continuing negative social norm in America.
   Answer: True

4. Segments of the community with the lowest socioeconomic status also have the poorest health and the most difficulty in gaining access to health care.
   Answer: True

5. Community organization is considered a science.
   Answer: False

6. In 1850, Lamuel Shattuck, drew up a health report for the Commonwealth of Massachusetts that outlined the public health needs of the state.
   Answer: True

7. In 1850, William Jenner drew up a health report for the Commonweatlh of Massachusetts that outlined the public health needs of the state.
   Answer: False

8. As the twentieth Century began, life expectancy in the U.S. was still less than 50 years.
   Answer: True

9. The Medicare and Medicaid bills passed by Congress in 1965 were amendments to the Social Security Act of 1935.
   Answer: True

10. Medicaid is a program that primarly assists in the payment of medical bills for the elderly.
    Answer: False

11. The 1970s, 1980s and 1990s have been characterized by repeated attempts and failures to bring the costs of health care under control.
    Answer: True

12. The 1979 United State Surgeon General's report, <u>Healthy People</u>, provided the basis for the nation's health plan for the 1980s.
    Answer: True

13. The leading causes of death in the United States today are communicable diseases.
    Answer: False

Essay

Write your answer in the space provided or on a separate sheet of paper.

1. Explain the difference between community health and public health.
   Answer: Community health includes both private and public efforts of individuals, groups, and organizations to promote, protect and preserve the health of those in the community while public health includes only the efforts of the government.

2. Explain how the economy affects the health of a community.
   Answer: An economic downturn means lower tax revenues for health and social services, and employers find it more difficult to provide health benefites for employees.

3. Name six social and cultural factors that affect the health of the community and give an example of each.
   Answer: beliefs, traditions and prejudices - the traditions of an ethnic group can impact the foods sold in a community economy - a drop in the economy usually indicates a drop in social services politics - the battle over universal health care religion - Jews not eating pork social norms - alcohol consumption in the U.S. socioeconomic status - those with the lowest socioeconomic status have the poorest health

4. Identify the major periods in the history of community and public health and give the approximate timeframe for each.
   Answer: Ancient Societies - before 500 B.C. Classical Cultures - 500 B.C. to 500 A.D. Middle Ages - 500 to 1500 A.D. Renaissance and Exploration - 1500 to 1700 A.D. eighteenth, nineteenth and twentieth Centuries - 1700 A.D. to present

5. Why is 1875 to 1900 known as the bacteriological period of public health?
   Answer: 1) Because of the work of Robert Koch who developed the criteria and procedures necessary to establish that a particular microbe, and no other, causes a particular disease, and 2) because of the identity of numerous bacterial disease agents was established.

6. What was the result of the National Hospital Survey and Construction Act of 1946?
   Answer: The rapid rate of hospital construction throughout the country between 1946 and 1960, with little thought given to health planning.

7. A study conducted by the Centers for Disease Control in 1975 on premature deaths indicated that 48% of all such deaths could be traced to one's lifestyle (health behavior). What kind of health behaviors were identified?
   Answer: Lifestyles characterized by a lack of exercise, high-fat diets, smoking, uncontrolled hypertension, and the inability to control stress were found to be contributing factors to premature mortality.

8. Identify the major health problems facing the people of the United States today.
   Answer: health care delivery, environmental problems, lifestyle diseases, communicable diseases, alcohol and other drug abuse

9. What is "Health for all by the year 2000"? What is the underlying concept of it? And, where was it first conceived?
   Answer: It is a target of the World Health Organization that the level of health to be attained by the turn of the century should be that which will permit all people to lead a socially and economically productive life. The underlying concept is that health resources should be distributed in such a way that essential health care services are accessible to everyone. This goal was first conceived at the 30th World Health Assembly of the World Health Organization in 1977.

10. What are the three broad goals of community health as expressesed in Healthy People 2000?
   Answer: To increase the span of healthy life of Americans To reduce health desparities among Americans To achieve access to preventive services for all Americans

Matching

Choose the item from Column 2 that best matches each item in Column 1.

Match the event in history with the appropriate date.

1. New Deal passed   1933

2. Clinton's health care plan released   1993

3. Founding of the American Cancer Society   1913

4. Social Security Act passed   1935

5. Medicaid and Medicaid enacted   1965

6. Years of Great Depression   1929-1935

7. Period of Social Engineering   1960-1975

8. School Health Education Study (SHES)   1962

9. year Healthy People was released   1979

10. Health For All By the Year 2000 was   1977
    conceived

Match the following activity with its proper classification.

11. choosing to eat wisely   personal health activity

12. protecting the food and water supply   community health activity

13. wearing a safety belt regularly   personal health activity

14. visiting a physician   personal health activity

15. raising money for the American Heart   community health activity
    Association

16. maintain accurate birth and death   community health activity
    records

Chapter 2   Organizations That Contribute to Community Health

Multiple-Choice

Choose the one alternative that best completes the statement or answers the question.

1. Official health agencies are financed primarily by:
   A) donations.
   B) tax dollars.
   C) voluntary giving.
   D) member dues.
   Answer: B

2. World Health Day is commemorated each year on April 7 because it was on that day in 1948 that the _____ officially began its work.
   A) Environmental Protection Agency
   B) International Red Cross
   C) World Health Organization
   Answer: C

3. The last known case of smallpox was diagnosed on October 26, 1977, in what country?
   A) Somalia
   B) Kenya
   C) Zaire
   D) Malawi
   Answer: A

4. The Public Health Service emerged in 1912 from:
   A) World Health Organization.
   B) Department of Health Education and Welfare.
   C) Marine Hospital Service.
   D) The Bethesda Naval Hospital.
   Answer: C

5. The research arm of the Public Health Service is the:
   A) Centers for Disease Control and Prevention.
   B) Health Resources and Services Administration.
   C) Agency for Toxic Substances and Disease Registry.
   D) National Institute of Health.
   Answer: D

6. The Food and Drug Administration sets health and safety standards for all:
   A) food.
   B) cosmetics.
   C) drugs.
   D) all of the above.
   E) just A and C.
   Answer: D

7. Which division of the Public Health Service has its purpose to improve the nation's health resources and services and their distribution to underserved populations?
   A) Centers for Disease Control and Prevention
   B) Health Resources and Services Administration
   C) National Institutes for Health
   D) Health Resources Administration
   Answer: B

8. Which division of the Public Health Service was created by Superfund legislation?
   A) Agency for Toxic Substances and Disease Registry
   B) Environmental Protection Agency
   C) Substance Abuse and Mental Health Services Administration
   D) Indian Health Service
   Answer: A

9. In most states, those eligible to head a local health department include:
   A) physicians and dentists.
   B) nurses.
   C) veterinarians and individuals with masters degrees in public health.
   D) A and B
   E) A and C
   Answer: E

10. The average person in a community receives most of his/her public health services from:
    A) Department of Health and Human Services.
    B) state health department.
    C) local health department.
    D) none of the above.
    Answer: C

11. Inspection of restaurants is the task of the:
    A) Food and Drug Administration.
    B) Department of Health and Human Services.
    C) state health department.
    D) local health department.
    Answer: D

12. Which of the following are quasi-official health organizations?
    A) WHO, FDA, and CDC
    B) American Cancer Society and American Heart Association
    C) American Red Cross and National Academy of Sciences
    D) American Lung Association and local health departments
    Answer: C

13. All of the following are non-governmental health agencies except:
    A) voluntary and professional agencies.
    B) local health departments.
    C) philanthropic and service agencies.
    D) religious agencies and corporations.
    Answer: B

14. At what levels do most voluntary health agencies exist?
    A) international, national, state, and local
    B) national, state, and local
    C) state and local
    Answer: B

15. Which philanthropic foundation is known for its support of the development of health maintenance organizations and community health promotion?
    A) Rockefeller Foundation
    B) Robert Wood Johnson Foundation
    C) Henry J. Kaiser Family Foundation
    D) W.K. Kellogg Foundation
    Answer: C

16. Which service organization has contributed greatly to the preservation of sight?
    A) Elks
    B) Lions
    C) Moose
    D) Jaycees
    Answer: B

17. Which groups have been especially useful in delivering health messages to the black American community?
    A) service
    B) voluntary health agencies
    C) philanthropic foundations
    D) religious
    Answer: D

18. The primary reason for corporate America's interest in community health is:
    A) lack of access to health care.
    B) rising cost of health care.
    C) the maldistribution of health care.
    D) the concern for national health insurance.
    Answer: B

True-False

Write T if the statement is true and F if the statement is false.

1. The most widely recognized international governmental health organization today is the World Health Organization.
   Answer: True

2. The most widely recognized international governmental health organization today is the United Nations' Children's Fund (UNICEF).
   Answer: False

3. The World Health Organization is the oldest international health organization.
   Answer: False

4. The Department of Health and Human Services was formed during the administration of President Gerald Ford in 1980.
Answer: False

5. The Secretary of the Department of Health and Human Services is appointed by the president and is a member of his/her cabinet.
Answer: True

6. The Surgeon General has responsibility for the Uniformed Public Health Service Officers.
Answer: True

7. Medicaid and Medicare are health insurance programs which are the responsibility of the Social Security Administration.
Answer: False

8. The head of the state health department is usually a medical doctor appointed by the governor.
Answer: True

9. In sparsely populated rural areas it is not uncommon to find more than one county served by a single health department.
Answer: True

10. Most people think of public schools as official health organizations.
Answer: False

11. The American Red Cross is funded with tax dollars.
Answer: False

12. The American Red Cross and the International Committee of the Red Cross are totally separate organizations.
Answer: True

13. Nongovernmental or unofficial health agencies are funded by private donations or, in some cases, by membership dues.
Answer: True

14. Voluntary health agencies are an American creation.
Answer: True

15. The sole purpose of the United Way is to raise money for community agencies.
Answer: False

16. It is not uncommon for professional health organizations to lobby to affect legislation in such a way as to benefit their membership and their profession.
Answer: True

Short Answer

Write the word or phrase that best completes each statement or answers the question.

1. In a sentence or two, state the primary objective of the World Health Organization.
   Answer: The primary objective of WHO as stated in its constitution is the attainment by all peoples of the best possible level of health.

2. How does the World Health Organization work to meet its objective?
   Answer: By providing two types of services to member nations: (1) providing funds to improve the health work force and to control specific diseases, and (2) by providing central technical services such as expert advisors, in some cases, on-the-scene technical service personnel.

3. What are the seven major divisions of the Public Health Service?
   Answer: The National Institutes for Health; Food and Drug Administration; Centers for Disease Control and Prevention; Health Resources and Services Administration; Indian Health Service; Agency for Toxic Substances and Disease Registry; and Substance Abuse and Mental Health Services Administration.

4. How does the state health department provide a link between federal and local health agencies?
   Answer: As (1) a conduit for federal funds (block grants) aimed at local health problems, and (2) the link between local needs and federal expertise.

5. What are the two official duties of the American Red Cross?
   Answer: (1) Acting as the official representative of the United States government during natural disasters, and (2) serving as the liaison between members of the actived armed forces and their families during emergencies.

6. List the basic objectives shared by all voluntary health agencies.
   Answer: (1) To raise money to fund research, (2) to provide education both to professionals and the public, and (3) to provide service to those individuals and families that are afflicted with the disease or health problem.

7. Why have religious groups been effective avenues for promoting health programs?
   Answer: They (1) have had a history of volunteerism and preexisting reinforcement contingencies for volunteerism, (2) can influence entire families, and (3) have accessible meeting room facilities.

Matching

Choose the item from Column 2 that best matches each item in Column 1.

Match the following organization with the type of agency.

1. National Science Foundation   quasi-official health agency

2. American Lung Association   unofficial health agency

3. World Health Organization   official health agency

4. American Public Health Association   unofficial health agency

5. National Academy of Sciences   quasi-official health agency

6. Department of Health and Human Services   official health agency

7. American Red Cross   quasi-official health agency

8. American Medical Association   unofficial health agency

9. state health department   official health agency

10. public schools   official health agency

Match the historic events with the correct year.

11. Founding of International Committee of   1863
    the Red Cross

12. Beginning of the American Cancer   1913
    Society

13. Marine Hospital Service formed   1798

14. Beginning of World Health Organization   1948

15. year of last case of smallpox   1977

16. founding of the Public Health Service   1912

Match the type of agency with the funding source.

17. state health departments   funded primarily by tax dollars

18. American Red Cross   funded primarily by donations

19. American Lung Association   funded primarily by donations

20. local health department   funded primarily by tax dollars

21. professional health organizations   funded primarily by member dues

22. American Cancer Society   funded primarily by donations

23. voluntary health agencies   funded primarily by donations

Chapter 3   Epidemiology: The Study of Disease, Injury, and Death in the Community

Multiple-Choice

Choose the one alternative that best completes the statement or answers the question.

1. Epidemiology has sometimes been referred to as:
   A) community medicine.
   B) health promotion and disease prevention.
   C) population medicine.
   D) community health.
   Answer: C

2. How many cases are required before a disease outbreak is considered an epidemic?
   A) 50 to 100 cases
   B) 1,000 cases
   C) 10% of the population
   D) depends upon the disease and the population
   Answer: D

3. What are diseases called that occur regularly in a population?
   A) epidemic diseases
   B) pandemic diseases
   C) endemic diseases
   D) regular diseases
   Answer: C

4. When both animals and humans are involved in a disease outbreak, which of the following is the appropriate term to describe it?
   A) endemic
   B) epidemic
   C) pandemic
   D) epizootic
   E) epizoodemic
   Answer: E

5. The term used to describe a widespread epidemic is:
   A) epizoodemic.
   B) endemic.
   C) pandemic.
   D) epizootic.
   Answer: C

6. Which man was responsible for interrupting the London Cholera Epidemic in 1849 by removing the pump handle from the Broad Street Pump?
   A) John Snow
   B) Louis Pasteur
   C) Walter Reed
   D) Benjamin Rush
   Answer: A

7. Which of the following are examples of acute diseases?
   A) common cold, influenza
   B) heart disease and cancer
   C) measles and mumps
   D) all of the above
   E) just A and C
   Answer: E

8. _____ is a special incidence rate calculated for a particular population for a single disease outbreak and expressed as a percent.
   A) Chronic rate
   B) Crude rate
   C) Attack rate
   D) Specific rate
   Answer: C

9. Crude death rates would be expected to be higher in a:
   A) younger population.
   B) older population.
   C) population with evenly distributed ages.
   Answer: B

10. Which of the following is a measure of the severity of a disease and is directly related to the virulence of the disease agent?
    A) crude death rate
    B) cause-specific mortality rate
    C) case fatality rate
    D) proportionate mortality ratio
    Answer: C

11. Which of the following is (are) a reason(s) local health departments receive notification of only 35% of the cases of some communicable diseases?
    A) Many physicians are not familiar with the requirement of reporting.
    B) Clinics may not report each and every case of a disease.
    C) Patients recover with or without treatment before a diagnosis is confirmed.
    D) all of the above
    E) none of the above
    Answer: D

12. All of the following are included in vital statistics _except_:
    A) births and deaths.
    B) notifiable diseases.
    C) marriages and divorces.
    D) infant deaths.
    Answer: B

13. The first U.S. Census was ordered in _____ for the purpose of apportioning representation to the House of Representatives.
    A) 1776
    B) 1790
    C) 1825
    D) 1875
    Answer: B

14. What type of epidemiological study is designed to answer the questions who, when and where?
    A) descriptive
    B) analytical
    C) experimental
    Answer: A

15. What type of epidemic curve illustrates the long-term trend of a disease?
    A) secular
    B) seasonal
    C) single epidemic
    Answer: A

16. Of the single epidemic curves, which would be best for charting a communicable disease?
    A) point source epidemic curve
    B) propagated epidemic curve
    C) neither of the above would be best
    Answer: B

17. What type of epidemiological study would be used to test hypotheses about relationships between health problems and possible risk factors?
    A) descriptive
    B) analytical
    C) experimental
    Answer: B

18. Retrospective (case/control) studies and prospective (cohort) studies are considered what type of epidemological studies?
    A) descriptive
    B) analytical
    C) experimental
    Answer: B

True-False

Write T if the statement is true and F if the statement is false.

1. An epizooliologist studies disease outbreaks in animals.
   Answer: True

2. The term used to describe a widespread epidemic is epizoodemic.
   Answer: False

3. The current outbreak of AIDS is an example of a pandemic.
   Answer: True

4. Incidence rates are calculated by dividing all current cases of a disease (old and new) by the total population.
   Answer: False

5. Prevalence rates are useful for the study of chronic disease.
   Answer: True

6. Crude rates can be misleading when populations differ in age structure or some other attribute.
   Answer: True

7. Incubation period can be defined as time between exposure to an infectious agent and the onset of symptoms.
   Answer: True

8. Retrospective studies almost never prove causation by themselves.
   Answer: True

9. Odds ratios are generated from prospective studies, while relative risks are generated from retrospective studies.
   Answer: False

10. The central feature of experimental studies is the control of variables surrounding the experimental subjects.
    Answer: True

11. Blindness refers to the practice in which neither the researcher nor subjects know who is receiving the treatment.
    Answer: False

Essay

Write your answer in the space provided or on a separate sheet of paper.

1. Define the term epidemiology.
   Answer: The study of the distribution and determinants of diseases and injuries in human populations.

136

2. What major epidemics were present during the years of 542 to 543, 1348 to 1349, 1793, 1849 and today?
   Answer: 542 to 543 and 1348 to 1349 (plague); 1793 (yellow fever); 1849 (cholera); today (AIDS).

3. Why are rates important to an epidemologist?
   Answer: Rates allow a comparison of outbreaks that occur at different times or in different places.

4. Given an estimated mid-year popluation of 50,000 for town x, 50 live births and 150 deaths, calculate the crude birth and death rates.
   Answer: crude birth rate = 150/50,000 x 1,000 = 3.0/1000; crude death rate = 50/50,000 x 1,000 = 1.0/1000.

5. Explain how the reporting of a death by a physician gets included in the final statistics released by the CDC.
   Answer: Physicians, clinics, and hospitals are required by law to report all births and deaths as well as all cases of certain notifiable diseases to their local health department (LHD). LHDs then are required by law to summarize all records and report them to their respective state health departments. State health departments summarize these reports and relay them to the CDC through the National Electronic Telecommunications System (NETS).

6. Name four sources of standardized national data that are available for community health workers.
   Answer: U.S. Census; Statistical Abstract of the United States; Monthly Vital Statistics Report; and Morbidity and Mortality Weekly Reports

7. Compare the advantages and disadvantates of retrospective and prospective studies.
   Answer: Retrospective - advantages - less expensive, completed quickly, useful in studying rare diseases - disadvantages - cannot determine true risk Prospective - advantages - can determine true risk - disadvantages - expensive, takes years to complete, hard to use with rare diseases

8. What are the four principles essential to properly designed experimental studies?
   Answer: (1) control of variables, (2) control groups, (3) randomization, (4) blindness.

Matching

Choose the item from Column 2 that best matches each item in Column 1.

Match the following rates with their synonyms.

1. natality rates   birth rates

2. morbidity rates   sickness rates

3. mortality rates   death rates

4. fatality rates   death rates

5. prevalence rates   current cases

6. incidence rates   new cases

Match the following terms with the appropriate type of study.

7. odds ratio   analytical

8. who, when, where   descriptive

9. control groups   experimental

10. retrospective   analytical

11. epidemic curve   descriptive

12. prospective   analytical

13. blindness   experimental

14. relative risk   analytical

15. double blind   experimental

16. placebos   experimental

Chapter 4 Epidemiology: Prevention and Control of Diseases and Health Conditions

Multiple-Choice

Choose the one alternative that best completes the statement or answers the question.

1. Which of the following are not biological causative agents?
    A) fungi and metazoa
    B) viruses and rickettsiae
    C) pesticides and food additives
    D) bacteria and protoza
    Answer: C

2. The process of lodgment and growth of a microorganism or virus in the host is called:
    A) infectious disease.
    B) communicable disease.
    C) infection.
    D) noncommunicable disease.
    Answer: C

3. Diseases or conditions in which symptoms continue longer than three months are referred to as:
    A) acute.
    B) communicable.
    C) chronic.
    D) noncommunicable.
    Answer: C

4. The ability of a biological agent to lodge and grow in a host is referred to as:
    A) pathogenicity.
    B) infectivity.
    C) infectious.
    D) communicable.
    Answer: B

5. What is the correct order of the chain of infection for transmission of a disease from one person to another?
    A) Establishment, portal of entry, transmission, portal of exit, reservior, pathogen.
    B) Pathogen, reservoir, protal of exit, transmission, portal of entry, establishment.
    C) Portal of exit, pathogen, reservoir, transmission, portal of entry, establishment.
    D) Reservoir, pathogen, portal of entry, transmission, portal of exit, establishment.
    Answer: B

6. Diseases for which the reservoir resides in animal populations are called:
    A) zoonoses.
    B) anthroponoses.
    C) epizootic.
    D) epizoodemic.
    Answer: A

7. Tuberculosis, influenza, hestoplasmosis, and legionellosis are examples of _ diseases.
   A) air-borne
   B) vehicle-borne
   C) vector-borne
   Answer: A

8. Place in order of cause of most deaths to least deaths, the three leading causes of death in the United States.
   A) coronary heart disease, cancer, stroke
   B) stroke, coronary heart disease, cancer
   C) malignant neoplasms, coronary artery disease, cerebrovscular disease
   Answer: A

9. Which cause of death in 1990 accounted for the greatest percentage of YPLL?
   A) unintentional injuries
   B) HIV/AIDS
   C) cancer
   D) stroke
   Answer: A

10. _____ is the early diagnosis and prompt treatment of diseases before the disease becomes advanced and disability becomes severe.
   A) Primary prevention
   B) Secondary prevention
   C) Tertiary prevention
   Answer: B

11. _____ is the limitation of freedom of movement of well persons or animals that have been exposed to a communicable disease until the incubation period has passed.
   A) Isolation
   B) Quarantine
   C) Disinfection
   Answer: B

12. When the HIV antibodies appear in the blood of an infected person this person is referred to as:
   A) HIV positive.
   B) HIV positive with AIDS.
   C) seropositive.
   D) either A and B.
   E) either A and C.
   Answer: E

13. Breast and testicular self-examinations, the hemocult test, and the Pap test are all examples of:
   A) tertiary prevention.
   B) secondary prevention.
   C) primary prevention.
   Answer: B

14. Which of the following is (are) modifiable risk factors?
    A) race and personality type
    B) gender and age
    C) basic metabolic rate
    D) smoking and lack of exercise
    Answer: D

True-False

Write T if the statement is true and F if the statement is false.

1. Heat and radiation are considered physical causative agents.
    Answer: True

2. Communicable diseases and infectious diseases mean the same thing.
    Answer: True

3. Transfer of a disease by touching, biting, kissing, and sexual intercourse are examples of indirect transmission.
    Answer: False

4. Biological transmission of communicable disease is much more important than mechanical transmission in terms of its impact on community health.
    Answer: True

5. By far, mosquitoes are the most important vectors of human disease.
    Answer: True

6. Stroke is the second leading cause of death in the United States.
    Answer: False

7. When parts of a neoplasm break off and are carried to other parts of the body, the cancer is said to have metastasized.
    Answer: True

8. Colon/rectum cancer is the leading cause of cancer deaths in both sexes.
    Answer: False

9. Smallpox is the only communicable disease that has been eradicated.
    Answer: True

10. Isolation and quarantine mean the same thing.
    Answer: False

11. Once a person is diagnosed as HIV positive with AIDS, death usually occurs within five years.
    Answer: True

12. According to the Universal Precaution guidelines, used needles are to be recapped before discarding.
    Answer: False

13. Morticians are also to follow Universal Precaution guidelines.
    Answer: True

14. Intervention following a heart attack or stroke is the lease effective and most expensive way to provide help to a cardiovascular disease patient.
    Answer: True

Essay

Write your answer in the space provided or on a separate sheet of paper.

1. Why is heart disease considered a multicausation disease?
   Answer: It has no single causative agent. Genetics, environmental factors such as stress, and behaviorioral choices, such as diet and exercise, all can contribute to heart disease.

2. Draw and label the simplifed communicable disease model.
   Answer: a triangle with one of these at each point - host, agent and environment

3. Draw and label the chain of infection.
   Answer: pathogen - reservoir - portal of exit - transmission - portal of entry - establishment of disease in new host

4. Draw and label the mullticausation disease model.
   Answer: Three circles (one inside of the other) with your genetic endowment in the center circle -your personality, beliefs, and behavioral choices in the middle circle -and economics, infectious disease outbreaks, water quality, air pollution, health care systems, environment in the outer circle.

5. List the five types of cardiovascular diseases (CVD) identified by the American Heart Association.
   Answer: coronary heart disease, hypertension, stroke, rheumatic heart disease, and congenital heart disease

6. Identify three criteria that could be used by a community when prioritizing prevention and control efforts.
   Answer: (1) The number of people who die from a disease, (2) the number of years of potential life lost (YPLL) attributable to a particular cause, and (3) the economic costs associated with a particular disease or health condition.

7. Calculate the years of potential life lost by the following individuals who died as a result of unintentional injuries. Ages: 5, 10, 15, 20, 25, 30, 35, 40, 45, 50, 55 and 60.
   Answer: 420 YPLL

8. Identify the major components of the Universal Precaution guidelines.
   Answer: (1) Use appropriate barriers (gloves, masks, eyewear, gowns), (2) wash hands and change gloves frequently, (3) dispose of all "sharps" appropriately.

Matching

Choose the item from Column 2 that best matches each item in Column 1.

Match the following diseases with the classification of the disease.

1. appendicitis   acute noncommunicable disease

2. coronary heart disease   chronic noncommunicable disease

3. AIDS   chronic communicable disease

4. chicken pox   acute communicable disease

5. diabetes   chronic noncommunicable disease

6. sprained ankles   acute noncommunicable disease

7. Lyme disease   chronic communicable disease

8. common cold   acute communicable disease

Match the following diseases with the transmitting vector.

9. malaria   transmitted by mosquitoes

10. Rocky Mountain spotted fever   transmitted by ticks

11. yellow fever   transmitted by mosquitoes

12. loaiasis   transmitted by flies

13. Lyme disease   transmitted by ticks

14. African sleeping sickness   transmitted by flies

Match the following prevention behaviors with the level of prevention.

15. breast self-examination   secondary prevention

16. personal hygiene   primary prevention

17. physical therapy   tertiary prevention

18. health education programs   primary prevention

19. immunizations   primary prevention

20. chlorination of the community's water   primary prevention
    supply

Chapter 5   Community Organization and Health Promotion Planning: Two Important Tools of Community Health

Multiple-Choice

Choose the one alternative that best completes the statement or answers the question.

1. _____ is intervention whereby individuals, groups and organizations engage in planned action to influence social problems. It is concerned with the enrichment, development, and/or change of social institutions.
   A) Community development
   B) Community organization
   C) Community effectiveness
   D) Community planning
   Answer: B

2. The Peace Corps is an example of what method of community organization?
   A) locality development
   B) social planning
   C) social action
   D) revolutionary techniques
   Answer: A

3. The United Way is an example of what method of community organization?
   A) locality development
   B) social planning
   C) social action
   D) revolutionary techniques
   Answer: B

4. The civil rights movement was an example of what method of community organization?
   A) social planning
   B) revolutionary techniques
   C) locality development
   D) social action
   Answer: D

5. If those who initiate community organization are members of the community, then the movement is referred to as being:
   A) grass-roots.
   B) top-down initiated.
   C) outside-in initiated.
   D) none of the above
   Answer: A

6. When community organization is initiated by individuals from outside of the community, the problem is said to be organized from the:
   A) bottom up.
   B) citizens.
   C) grass-roots.
   D) top down.
   Answer: D

7. Community gatekeepers could include which of the following?
   A) politicians
   B) clergy
   C) business and education leaders
   D) all the above
   E) none of the above
   Answer: D

8. When the top-down approach to community organization is being used, organizers might find it advantageous to enter the community through:
   A) the city council.
   B) a group of elected officials.
   C) a well-respected organization or institution that is already in the community.
   D) the Board of Education.
   Answer: C

9. When organizing people to solve a community problem, it is best to begin with:
   A) those causing the problem.
   B) a good group of volunteers.
   C) the victims of similar problems.
   D) those who are already interested in seeing that the problem be solved.
   Answer: D

10. The core group of any organized effort are also known as:
    A) executive participants.
    B) volunteers.
    C) a coalition.
    D) an association.
    Answer: A

11. Which of the following can be defined as a temporary union of two or more individuals and/or organizations to achieve a common purpose (often, to compensate for deficits in power, resources and expertise)?
    A) association
    B) task force
    C) coalition
    D) ad hoc committee
    Answer: C

12. Which of the following is a term used to delineate the real problem of a community?
    A) need assessment
    B) community analysis
    C) community diagnois
    D) all of the above
    E) none of the above
    Answer: D

13. Which of the following best describes the relationship between health education and health promotion/disease prevention?
    A) The terms mean the same thing.
    B) HP/DP is much more encompassing than health education.
    C) HP/DP is an important component of health education.
    D) None of the above are true.
    Answer: B

14. The best known and most often used health promotion planning model is the:
    A) PRECEDE/PROCEED.
    B) Model for Health Education Planning.
    C) Model for the Analysis of Health Education Planning and Resource Development.
    D) Comprehensive Health Education Model.
    E) Generic Health/Fitness Delivery System.
    Answer: A

15. Those whom the HP/DP program is intended to serve are known as the:
    A) coalition.
    B) target population.
    C) executive participants.
    D) stakeholders.
    Answer: B

16. Target population needs as seen through the eyes of the program planners are referred to as:
    A) service needs or real needs.
    B) service demand or wants.
    C) perceived or felt needs.
    Answer: A

17. The importance of an unmet need, how changeable the need is, and whether adequate resources are available to meet the need are all helpful in_ needs.
    A) explaining
    B) prioritizing
    C) validating
    D) determining
    Answer: B

18. To help employees learn how to manage their stress is an example of a program:
    A) purpose.
    B) goal.
    C) objective.
    D) all the above
    E) none of the above
    Answer: B

19. Intervention activities aimed at groups are referred to as:
    A) macro intervention activities.
    B) micro intervention activities.
    C) community based activities.
    D) health promotion/disease prevention activities.
    Answer: A

20. When implementing a HP/DP program, which of the following is not advised?
    A) Pilot test the program with people not like those in the target population.
    B) Pilot test it first.
    C) If a major flaw is found in pilot testing it should be re-piloted.
    D) Phase in the program.
    Answer: A

21. Mandates, values, norms, and comparison groups are examples of:
    A) formative evaluation.
    B) summative evaluation.
    C) standards of acceptibility.
    D) categories of objectives.
    Answer: C

22. _____ begins with the development of goals and objectives and is conducted after implementation to determine the impact of the program on the target population.
    A) Process evaluation
    B) Summative evaluation
    C) Formative evaluation
    D) none of the above
    Answer: B

23. Which of the mini-steps of program evaluation includes selecting an evaluator, identifying an evaluation design, and creating a timeline for the evaluation?
    A) planning the evaluation
    B) collecting the data
    C) analyzing the data
    D) reporting the results
    E) applying the results
    Answer: A

148

True-False

Write T if the statement is true and F if the statement is false.

1. Community organization is not a science but an art of consensus-building within a democratic process.
   Answer: True

2. Changes in community living that are self-imposed or self-developed have a meaning and permanence that imposed changes do not have.
   Answer: True

3. Gatekeepers are those who control, both formally and informally, the political climate of the community.
   Answer: True

4. Over the last 30 years, the number of people in many communities interested in volunteering their time has increased.
   Answer: False

5. There are fewer single-parent households today than there were 20 years ago.
   Answer: False

6. Most community problems are complex and the reality is that someone usually benefits if a problem remains unsolved.
   Answer: True

7. When conducting a needs assessment, great care must be taken to assure that collected data are both representative and unbiased.
   Answer: True

8. When prioritizing identified problems, it is important for general agreement or consensus to be used in order for ownership to take hold.
   Answer: True

9. It is not uncommon to have turf struggles when trying to build consensus.
   Answer: True

10. Healthy People 2000 is a publication that presents the health goals and objectives of the United States for the year 2000.
    Answer: True

11. Most people change their behavior based upon a single exposure (dose).
    Answer: False

12. "Hitting" the target population from several angles or through multiple channels should increase the chances of making an impact.
    Answer: True

13. Dosage is important in helping to change behavior.
    Answer: True

14. A pilot test can be thought of as a trial run.
    Answer: True

Essay

Write your answer in the space provided or on a separate sheet of paper.

1. List, in order of occurance, the 10 steps in the generalized approach to community organization.
   Answer: (1) recognition of a problem; (2) gaining entry into the community; (3) organizing the people; (4) identifying the specific problem; (5) determining priorities and setting goals; (6) arriving at a solution and selecting intervention activities; (7) implementation; (8) evaluation; (9) maintaining the outcomes over time; (10) looping back

2. Identify five things community organizers should consider when expanding their constituencies.
   Answer: (1) Identify people who are impacted by the problem that they are trying to solve; (2) provide "perks" or otherwise reward volunteers; (3) keep volunteer time short; (4) match volunteer assignments with the ability and expertise of the volunteers; and (5) consider providing appropriate training to make sure volunteers are comfortable with their tasks.

3. List the five steps of the needs assessment process and give an example of each step using the health problem of smoking.
   Answer: (1) Determing the present state of health of the target population. Example: How much smoking related morbidity and mortality exist in the target populaiton: What percent of the target population smoke? (2) Identifying existing programs. Example: Are there smoking cessation efforts presently in place in the community? (3) Comparing health deficits with existing programs. Example: What are the unmet needs related to smoking cessation? (4) Dealing with the problems. Example: The problem could be best handled through smoking cessation and school health education programs. (5)

4. What are the differences between goals and objectives?
   Answer: Goals (1) are much more encompassing and global, (2) are written to cover all aspects of a program, (3) provide overall program direction, (4) are more general in nature, (5) usually take longer to complete, (6) are usually not observed but inferred, and (7) often not easily measured.

5. Present, in order, the hierarchy of program objectives.
   Answer: Awareness, knowledge, attitudes, skills, access to health, behavior change, risk reduction, and health status.

Matching

Choose the item from Column 2 that best matches each item in Column 1.

Match the following activities with the type of community organization effort.

1. gay rights march   social action

2. United Way   social planning

3. Peace Corp   locality development

4. civil rights movement   social action

5. political oppression   revolutionary techniques

Match the following descriptions with the appropriate type of statement.

6. are more precise   objectives

7. usually take longer to complete   goals

8. are more general in nature   goals

9. observable and measurable   objectives

10. provide overall program direction   goals

11. more global   goals

Chapter 6   The School Health Program: A Component of Community Health

Multiple-Choice

Choose the one alternative that best completes the statement or answers the question.

1. A comprehensive school health program should include but not be limited to:
    A) health services, healthful school living, and health education.
    B) food service and social work.
    C) psychological services, and employee health promotion.
    D) all the above
    Answer: D

2. Less than _____ percent of the school districts in the United States have comprehenisve school health programs.
    A) 1
    B) 2
    C) 3
    D) 4
    E) 5
    Answer: E

3. The primary role of the school health team is to:
    A) plan the health education ourriculum.
    B) support the work of the school nurse.
    C) ensure the safety of all children.
    D) provide coordination of the various components of the comprehensive school health program.
    Answer: D

4. Which individuals are most often selected to serve as the coordinator of the school health team?
    A) counseling personnel or social workers
    B) physical educators or parents
    C) health educators or school nurses
    D) none of the above
    Answer: C

5. Which of the following is not true about school nurses?
    A) Is in a position to provide leadership for the school health program.
    B) Could be employed by either a school district or local health department.
    C) Has the primary responsibility of providing first aid for students.
    D) Has the responsibility to construct and/or maintain school health records for students.
    Answer: C

6. It is not uncommon for an elementary school teacher to:
   A) be responsible for the school health program.
   B) spend more waking hours with students than the parents spend with their children.
   C) be responsible for maintaining school health records.
   D) identify community resources for school health services.
   Answer: A

7. According to the Association for the Advancement of Health Education, the school nurse should:
   A) have state licensure as a registered professional nurse.
   B) hold a baccalaureate degree.
   C) have studied health education.
   D) all of the above
   E) just A and B
   Answer: D

8. Which of the following is not true about school health policies (SHPs)?
   A) SHPs guide all those who work in the program.
   B) SHPs describe the nature of the program to those outside the program.
   C) SHPs are comprised primarily of first aid procedures.
   D) SHPs provide a means of accountability for the school health program.
   Answer: C

9. Which of the following people should approve school health policies?
   A) the school districts medical advisor
   B) the school administration
   C) the board of education
   D) all the above should approve the policies
   Answer: D

10. _____ is (are) that part of the school health program provided by physicians, nurses, dentists, health educators, other allied health personnel, social workers, teachers and others to appraise, protect and promote the health of students and school personnel.
    A) Administration and organization
    B) School health services
    C) Healthful school environment
    D) Health instruction
    Answer: B

11. Which model of school health services includes a school based clinic?
    A) basic health services
    B) expanded health services
    C) comprehensive health services
    D) both A and C
    Answer: C

12. The responsibility for maintaining a safe school environment should rest with:
    A) the school board.
    B) the police.
    C) all who use it.
    D) teachers and administrators.
    Answer: C

13. Which method of instruction allows for the greatest opportunity for a sequential program arranged to consider the needs, interests, and developmental levels of the students?
    A) direct instruction
    B) correlated instruction
    C) integratial instruction
    Answer: A

14. The National Diffussion Network helps school personnel to:
    A) write health curricula.
    B) select appropriate curricular materials.
    C) rate their own curricula.
    D) none of the above
    Answer: B

15. The one comprehensive health curriculium found in the National Diffusion Network list is:
    A) Growing Healthy.
    B) Teenage Health Teaching Modules.
    C) Teenage Health Teaching Modules.
    D) School Health Education Study.
    Answer: A

16. Which of the following curricula can stand alone as a curriculum or supplement other curricular materials?
    A) Have a Healthy Heart
    B) School Health Education Study
    C) Teenage Health Teaching Modules
    D) Adolescent Health Guide
    Answer: C

17. Which of the following curricula was developed as a compatible curriculium for Growing Healthy?
    A) Have a Healthy Heart
    B) School Health Eduction Study
    C) Teenage Health Teaching Modules
    D) Adolescent Health Guide
    Answer: C

18. School districts could help reduce controversy by:
    A) using acceptable teaching methods.
    B) making sure qualifed and interested teachers teach health.
    C) implementing age-appropriate curricula.
    D) all the above
    E) none of the above
    Answer: D

19. Most of the controversy surrounding SBCs/SLCs has centered on the issue of:
    A) using tax dollars.
    B) reproductive health care.
    C) taking work away from private health providers.
    D) too costly.
    Answer: B

True-False

Write T if the statement is true and F if the statement is false.

1. Less than 2% of the school districts in the United States have comprehensive school health programs.
   Answer: False

2. It is not unusual for there to be a lack of coordination among school employees regarding the components of a school health program.
   Answer: True

3. Teachers are in a position to make judgments on the "normal and abnormal" behavior of students.
   Answer: True

4. Health of children and their learning are reciprocally related.
   Answer: True

5. At the present time, approximately one-half of the states and territories in the United States have school districts that employ school health coordinators.
   Answer: True

6. By law, school districts are required to provide a safe school environment.
   Answer: True

7. Health instruction and school health education mean the same thing.
   Answer: False

8. School health education can take place when the school nurse gives a vision screening test to a student.
   Answer: True

9. The scope of a curriculum outlines when content will be taught.
   Answer: False

10. The sequence of a curriculum outlines what will be taught.
    Answer: False

11. Growing Healthy is a comprehensive health curriculum designed for grades K to 12.
    Answer: False

12. A number of health agencies and organizations produce curricula for use in K-6.
    Answer: True

13. The majority of school-based clinic/school-linked clinics have functioned as primary care providers for medically underserved adolescents.
Answer: True

14. School-based clinics/school-linked clinics have been the frequent targets of intense criticism at the local and national levels by political and religious groups.
Answer: True

Essay

Write your answer in the space provided or on a separate sheet of paper.

1. Why do school health programs have great potential for impacting the health of the nation.
Answer: (1) Numbers. There are 46 million school-age children children and 5 million school employees, (2) school attendance is required.

2. In what areas of the school health program can each of the following people best contribute to comprehensive school health: school nurse, health education, and maintenance workers?
Answer: School nurse (health services), health educators (health eduation), maintenance workers (healthful school environment).

3. If you were going to create a school health team who would be in it and why?
Answer: Adminstrators, food service workers, counseling personnel, maintenance workers, medical personnel, social workers, parents, students, teachers, and representatives from appropriate community agencies.

4. What impact can the School Breakfast Program (SBP) have on the students who participate?
Answer: Research shows that students who participate in SBP enhanced their abilities to learn compared to those who do not. Beyond the educational benefits, SBP participation has also improved total daily nutrient intake and nutritional status, shown to help control body weight by minimizing compulsive eating, and possibly reducing risk of coronary heart disease by lowering blood cholesterol.

5. What are the advantages of having school health services as a means of delivering health care?
Answer: (1) equitability, (2) breadth of coverage, (3) confidentiality, (4) user friendly, and (5) convenience

6. Besides scope and sequence, what are the components commonly found in a school curriculum?
Answer: (1) objective, (2) learning activities, (3) possible instructional resources, and (4) methods for determining the extent to which the objectives are met.

7. Identify three major challenges that still face those who work in school health and state why they are challenges.
Answer: (1) comprehensive school health -few schools have it, (2) dealing with conservative groups and the concern about teaching values and open-ended decision making, and (3) school-based clinics or school-linked clinics -reproductive health issues

Matching

Choose the item from Column 2 that best matches each item in Column 1.

Match the following elements of school health with the appropriate school health component.

1. school health coordinator   administration and organization

2. emergency care   school health services

3. physical plant   healthful school environment

4. physical environment   healthful school environment

5. curriculum   health instruction

6. social/emotional environment   healthful school enivronment

7. scope   health instruction

8. health appraisals   school health services

9. sequence   health instruction

10. prevention and control of communicable diseases   school health services

11. school violence   healthful school environment

12. school health education   health instruction

Match the following descriptions with the type of instruction.

13. requires much coordination with others   correlated instruction

14. separate subject   direct instruction

15. major emphasis on special subject area not health   integrated instruction

16. taught with other subjects   correlated instruction

17. uses health as a vehicle to teach other material   integrated instruction

18. method preferred by school health advocates   direct instruction

Match the following events with the appropriate health education curriculum.

19. began in 1960   School Health Education Study

20. developed for K-6   Growing Healthy

21. comprehensive curriculum on NDN list   Growing Healthy

22. contains aerobic activity component   Have a Healthy Heart

23. developed for 7-12   Teenage Health Teaching Modules

24. resulted from the combination of the   Growing Healthy
    School Health Curriculm Project and the
    Primary Grades Health Curriculum
    Project.

Chapter 7   A Health Profile of the American People

Multiple-Choice

Choose the one alternative that best completes the statement or answers the question.

1. Forty to 70% of all premature deaths, one-third of all acute disabilities, and two-thirds of all chronic disabilities could be elimnated if Americans:
   B) lived in a cleaner environment.
   C) maintained a regular exercise routine.
   D) had better health behavior.
   Answer: D

2. Most measures of health and health status are based on:
   A) unrealiable numbers.
   B) ill health and death.
   C) births and deaths.
   D) voluntary health agency data.
   Answer: B

3. The most accurate and easily acquired health data are those for:
   A) morbidity.
   B) fertility.
   C) mortality.
   D) births.
   Answer: C

4. The most reliable single indicator of health status of a population is:
   A) birth.
   B) death.
   C) illness.
   D) sickness.
   Answer: B

5. The leading causes of death in the United States in the early 1900s were:
   A) heart disease and cancer.
   B) communicable diseases.
   C) noninfectious diseases.
   D) noncommunicable diseases.
   Answer: B

6. In the 1990s, what percent of all deaths are caused by the four leading causes of death -heart disease, cancer, strokes and unintentional injuries?
   A) 66 to 75%
   B) 45 to 55%
   C) 30 to 40%
   D) 10 to 15%
   Answer: A

7. The country with the highest life expectancy is:
   A) England.
   B) Germany.
   C) United States.
   D) Japan.
   Answer: D

8. The country with the lowest life expectancy are those:
   A) of the middle East.
   B) with weakly developed economies.
   C) with well-developed economies.
   D) those closest to the equator.
   Answer: B

9. A premature death is any death prior to:
   A) retirement.
   B) receiving social security.
   C) age 55.
   D) age 65.
   Answer: D

10. The greatest number of YPLL for the population as a whole are the result of:
    A) heart disease and cancer.
    B) heart disease and stroke.
    C) unintentional injuries and cancer.
    D) unintentional injuries and heart disease.
    Answer: C

11. Which of the following is not true?
    A) In general, young assess their health better than old do.
    B) In general, males assess their health better than females do.
    C) In general, blacks assess their health better than whites do.
    D) All the above are true.
    Answer: C

12. Homicides and suicides are great concerns in which cohort(s)?
    A) infants
    B) children
    C) adolescents and young adults
    D) adults
    E) older adults
    Answer: C

13. Which childhood disease made a resurgence in the late 1980s and impacted many adolescents and young adults?
    A) mumps
    B) measles
    C) whooping cough
    D) polio
    E) chicken pox
    Answer: B

162

14. Which of the following includes national school-based surveys, state and local-based surveys, and a national household-based survey?
    A) National Health Interview Survey
    B) National Health and Nutrition Examination Survey
    C) Youth Risk Behavior Surveillance System
    D) DALYs
    Answer: C

15. The most popular illicit drug among adolescents and young adults in recent years has been:
    A) alcohol.
    B) LSD.
    C) marijuana.
    D) crack cocaine.
    Answer: C

16. Teenage mothers are:
    A) less likely to complete high school.
    B) more likely to be unemployed.
    C) more likely to lack parenting skills.
    D) all the above
    E) just A and B
    Answer: D

17. The leading cause of cancer deaths and the most preventable type of cancer for both men and women is:
    A) colorectal.
    B) lung.
    C) skin.
    D) stomach.
    Answer: B

18. Eighty-five percent of all lung cancer deaths can be attributed to:
    A) the environment.
    B) smoking.
    C) living in a polluted area.
    D) heredity.
    Answer: B

19. In general, smoking rates are higher among:
    A) blacks and Hispanics than whites.
    B) blue-collar workers than white-collar workers.
    C) people with fewer years of education.
    D) all the above
    E) just A and B
    Answer: D

20. Being overweight increases ones chances of all the following <u>except</u>:
    A) gall bladder disease.
    B) heart disease.
    C) sickle cell anemia.
    D) some cancers.
    Answer: C

21. The most prevalent cardiovascular disease is:
    A) hypertension.
    B) stroke.
    C) heart attack.
    D) none of the above
    Answer: A

22. The fastest growing segment of the senior population are those who are:
    A) 65+ years old.
    B) 70+ years old.
    C) 75+ years old.
    D) 85+ years old.
    Answer: D

23. Which of the following is not a chronic condition of seniors?
    A) heart disease
    B) cataracts
    C) diabetes
    D) emphysemia
    Answer: B

True-False

Write T if the statement is true and F if the statement is false.

1. It is difficult to measure how much health exists in a given population.
   Answer: True

2. The leading causes of death in the United States in the early 1900s were noncommunicable diseases.
   Answer: False

3. Life expectancy is usually a pretty good predictor of how long any one person will live.
   Answer: False

4. Most Americans believe they are in good, very good, or excellent health.
   Answer: True

5. Alcohol and drugs are involved in over half of all homicides.
   Answer: True

6. Measles is a much more severe disease for adolescents and young adults than it is for children.
   Answer: True

7. The use of <u>smokable</u> tobacco by adolescents and young adults in recent years is on the rise as measured by per capita consumption.
   Answer: False

8. The use of <u>smokeless</u> tobacco by adolescents and young adults in recent years is on the rise.
   Answer: True

9. The number of cases of breast cancer is twice that of lung cancer in women.
   Answer: True

10. Light to moderate physical activity can have significant health benefits.
    Answer: True

11. The most prevalent cardiovascular disease is stroke.
    Answer: False

12. Once detected, hypertension is a risk factor that is highly modifiable.
    Answer: True

13. Life expectancy of those reaching the age of 65 years has consistently decreased since 1900.
    Answer: False

Essay

Write your answer in the space provided or on a separate sheet of paper.

1. Why has there been a shift in the leading causes of death in the early 1900s from communicable disease to the noncommunicable diseases of today?
   Answer: Because of the progress in public health practice and biomedical research.

2. State what you feel to be the best single measure of health status and provide a rationale for your choice.
   Answer: There is no best answer!

3. Identify and name the five age groups of Americans recognized by the United States government and note a major health problem of each.
   Answer: infants - infant mortality, mother's behavior during pregnancy children - childhood diseases, social morbidities adolescents and young adults - homicide and suicide, motor vehicle crashes adults - illness and death from lifestyle older adults - chronic conditions, impairments

Matching

Choose the item from Column 2 that best matches each item in Column 1.

Match the following descriptions with the different measures of health status.

1. unintentional injuries is the leading cause of _____ in men

   years of potential life lost

2. longer for women then men

   life expectancy

3. based on self report

   National Health Interview Survey

4. based on clinical testing

   National Health and Nutrition Examination Survey

5. highest in Japan

   life expectancy

6. includes mortality and disability

   disability-adjusted life years

7. determined by subtracting death age from 65

   years of potential life lost

8. heart disease leads the way today

   mortality

9. cancer is the leading cause in women

   years of potential life lost

10. longer for whites than blacks

    life expectancy

11. DALYs

    disability-adjusted Life Years

12. NHANES

    National Health and Nutritional Examination Survey

Match the following health concerns with the appropriate classification of Americans.

13. judge of parenting skills

    child (1 to 14 years) health

14. pneumonia is a leading cause of death

    older adult (65 + years) health

15. whooping cough, diphtheria

    child (1 to 14 years) health

16. homicide and suicide deaths

    adolescent and young adult (15 to 24 years) health

17. hypertension defined as 160/90

    older adult (65 + years) health

18. measles, polio

    children (1 to 14 years) health

19. cancer leading cause of death

    adult (25 to 64 years) health

166

20. motor vehicle crash deaths	adolescent and young adult (15 to 24 years) health
21. smokeless tobacco use on the rise	adolescent and young adult (15 to 24 years) health
22. best judge of a nation's health	infant (< 1 year old) health
23. cataracts	older adult (65+ years) health
24. hearing impairments	older adult (65+ years) health

Chapter 8   Maternal, Infant, and Child Health

Multiple-Choice

Choose the one alternative that best completes the statement or answers the question.

1. Maternal health is regarded as the health of a women of child-bearing age during which of the following times?
    A) pre-pregnancy and pregnancy
    B) labor and delivery
    C) postpartal
    D) all the above
    E) just A and B
    Answer: D

2. The primary drop in the maternal mortality rate in the United States from 1970 to 1990 is:
    A) the increased number of physicians.
    B) new screening procedures.
    C) high-technology equipment.
    D) better access to health care.
    E) B and C
    Answer: E

3. Maternal mortality rate was _____ times higher for black Americans than white Americans.
    A) 2
    B) 4
    C) 6
    D) 10
    Answer: B

4. The two primary risk factors of maternal morbidity and mortality are:
    A) use of alcohol and poor nutrition.
    B) lack of prenatal care and teenage pregnancy.
    C) lack of exercise and good health care.
    D) none of the above
    Answer: B

5. The average cost of prenatal care in the United States in 1993 was:
    A) $500.
    B) $700.
    C) $1000.
    D) $1500.
    Answer: B

6. One out of every _____ teenage females in the United States became pregnant in 1993.
   A) 5
   B) 10
   C) 15
   D) 20
   Answer: B

7. Teenage pregnancy means:
   A) greater health risks for mother and child.
   B) the mother is more likely to experience an early divorce if she marries.
   C) the mother is less likely to attain an adequate education than her nonpregnant counter part.
   D) all the above
   E) just A and C
   Answer: D

8. The death of a child during the first 28 days after birth is called:
   A) infant death.
   B) neonatal death.
   C) postneonatal death.
   D) fetal death.
   Answer: B

9. The death of a child between the age of 28 and 365 days is called:
   A) infant death.
   B) neonatal death.
   C) postneonatal death.
   D) fetal death.
   Answer: C

10. The country with the lowest infant mortality rate in the world is:
    A) Japan.
    B) United States.
    C) Sweden.
    D) Canada.
    Answer: A

11. A premature infant is one born:
    A) following a gestation period of 38 weeks or less.
    B) at a low birth weight.
    C) to a teenage mother.
    D) all the above
    E) just A and B
    Answer: E

12. Sudden Infant Death Syndrome usually occurs between the ages of
    A) birth and one year.
    B) birth and two months.
    C) 2 and 4 months.
    D) 6 months to a year.
    Answer: C

170

13. In 1988, the "gag rule" was enacted to:
    A) allow personnel in public family planning clinics to discuss abortion with clients.
    B) prohibit the discussion of contraception in public health clinics.
    C) allow personnel to discuss contraception in public health clinics.
    D) ban physicians and nurses in clinics receiving federal funds from counseling clients about abortions.
    Answer: D

14. Approximately what percent of abortions in the United States are performed on teenagers?
    A) 10
    B) 25
    C) 40
    D) 50
    Answer: B

15. Approximately what percent of unmarried and teenage mothers receive either late or no prenatal care?
    A) 10
    B) 25
    C) 50
    D) 75
    Answer: C

16. Those women who have no prenatal care and show up at a health care facility to give birth are called:
    A) last minute deliveries.
    B) drop-in deliveries.
    C) no show deliveries.
    D) no care deliveries.
    Answer: B

17. The Special Supplemental Food Program for Women, Infants, and Children (WIC) is sponsored by:
    A) U.S. Department of Health and Human Services.
    B) U.S. Department of Agriculture.
    C) Centers for Disease Control and Prevention.
    D) Public Health Service.
    Answer: B

18. Studies have shown that the WIC program has produced a cost benefit ratio of:
    A) 1:2.
    B) 1:3.
    C) 1:5.
    D) 1:10.
    Answer: B

19. The Family and Medical Leave Act that went into effect in 1993 excludes about what percent of American employees?
    A) 20
    B) 40
    C) 60
    D) 80
    Answer: B

20. The Family and Medical Leave Act covers employees:
    A) after the birth of a child.
    B) after an adoption.
    C) in the event of illness in the immediate family.
    D) all the above
    E) just A and B
    Answer: D

True-False

Write T if the statement is true and F if the statement is false.

1. Maternal health encompasses the health of women in child-bearing age from pre-pregnancy through pregnancy, labor and delivery, and the postpartal period.
   Answer: True

2. Maternal health in the United States in the last 20 years has improved steadily.
   Answer: True

3. By definition, prenatal health care is the medical care received by the pregnant woman from the time of conception until the birth process occurs.
   Answer: True

4. The United States has one of the lowest teenage pregnancy rates of any developed country in the world.
   Answer: False

5. A neonatologist is a medical doctor who specializes in the care of newborn children up to two months of age.
   Answer: True

6. Deaths in utero with a gestational age of at least 20 weeks are called neonatal deaths.
   Answer: False

7. The United States has one of the lowest infant mortality rates of any of the developed countries in the world.
   Answer: False

8. A safe level of alcohol consumption during pregnancy has not been determined.
   Answer: True

9. The exact cause of Sudden Infant Death Syndrome is unknown.
   Answer: True

10. The United States' system for immunizing children against childhood disease is very efficient in seeing that the children get immunized on time.
    Answer: False

11. Family planning can be defined as determing the preferred number and spacing of children and choosing the appropriate means to achieve this preference.
    Answer: True

12. Title X of the Public Health Service Act was established in 1970 to provide family planning services to low-income people.
    Answer: True

13. President Bush lifted the "gag rule" regulations in 1988.
    Answer: False

14. The majority of women who receive abortions are single, white, and qualify for welfare.
    Answer: True

15. One of the drawbacks of categorically funded health programs is that some needy people "fall through the cracks" and are not served.
    Answer: True

16. All but two states in the United States require evidence of vaccination before a child may enter school.
    Answer: False

17. There is a new vaccine, Tetramune, that reduces the number of injections a child will need to be immunized properly.
    Answer: True

18. The United States is the only industrialized nation that has not enacted a paid infant care leave act.
    Answer: True

19. The children most likely to receive inadequate child care are the children of working lower and middle class families.
    Answer: True

Essay

Write your answer in the space provided or on a separate sheet of paper.

1. Calculate the maternal mortality rate for the following: A. 29 deaths for 100,000 live births; B. 15 deaths for 50,000 live births.
   Answer: A. 29/100,000; B. 30/100,000

2. What are the risks for babies born to teenage mothers?
   Answer: (1) Low birth weight, (2) prematurity, (3) lower IQ scores, and (4) higher mortality
   rates.

3. What factors have contributed to the lowering of the infant mortality rate in the United
   States?
   Answer: (1) improvements in socioeconomic status, (2) housing, (3) nutrition, (4) levels of
   immunization, (5) availability of clean water, pasteurized milk, and antibotics, and
   (6) modern medical technology.

4. Briefly describe Fetal Alcohol Syndrome (FAS) and Sudden Infant Death Syndrome (SIDS).
   Answer: FAS - A term used to describe a group of defects in babies born to mothers who have
   consumed high levels of alcohol during pregnancy; can lead to growth and mental
   retardation. SIDS - Sudden unanticipated death of an infant in whom, after
   examination, there is no recognized cause of death. Usually occurs in infants between
   the ages of 2 - 4 months.

5. Briefly describe the criteria for women, infants and children to be eligible for WIC.
   Answer: (1) Reside in the state in which they are applying for the WIC program, (2) meet the
   income guideline, and (3) meet the nutritional risk criteria as determined by a
   medical and/or nutritional assessment.

6. Why do children still get childhood diseases when immunizations exist to prevent them?
   Answer: (1) Approximately 2% of the children enter school without being properly immunized,
   (2) even when properly administered, immunizations have a failure rate of between 2
   and 5%, (3) about 5% of students are given religious and medical exemptions from
   immunization requirements, and (4) one-third of preschoolers in the U.S. have not been
   immunized properly.

Matching

Choose the item from Column 2 that best matches each item in Column 1.

Match the following descriptions with the chance of receiving prenatal care.

1.	well-educated women	more likely to receive prenatal health care
2.	women already with children	less likely to receive prenatal health care
3.	white women	more likely to receive prenatal care
4.	women living in poverty	less likely to receive prenatal health care
5.	Native Americans	less likely to receive prenatal health care
6.	married women	more likely to receive prenatal health care
7.	experience with the health care system	more likely to receive prenatal health care
8.	those who speak English	more likely to receive prenatal care

Match the following descriptions with the possible outcome.

9. environmental hazards

cause of many birth defects

10. smoking

maternal risk factor associated with giving birth to a low-birth-weight infant

11. domestic violence

primary cause of childhood morbidity

12. poverty

maternal risk factor associated with giving birth to a low-birth-weight infant

13. educational status

maternal risk factor associated with giving birth to a low-birth-weight infant

14. unintentional injuries

primary cause of childhood morbidity

15. neglect

primary cause of childhood morbidity

16. giving birth prior to age 17 or after 40

maternal risk factor associated with giving birth to a low-birth-weight infant

Match the following descriptions with items related to the issue of abortion.

17. made it illegal to use Federal funds for abortions

Hyde Amendment of 1976

18. believe life begins at conception

Pro-life

19. unborn child has no rights under the law

Roe vs. Wade

20. women have a right to reproductive freedom

Pro-choice

21. ruling that made it unconstitutional for state laws to prohibit abortions

Roe vs. Wade

22. reduced the number of white babies available for adoption

Roe vs. Wade

Chapter 9   Community Health and Minorities

Multiple-Choice

Choose the one alternative that best completes the statement or answers the question.

1. The majority of people living in the United States are white. Approximately what percent of the population falls into this classification?
   A) 50
   B) 60
   C) 70
   D) 80
   Answer: D

2. According to the Office of Management and Budget Directive 15 titled "Race and Ethnic Standards for Federal Statistics and Administrative Reporting" which of the following is not considered a race?
   A) American Indian or Alaskan Native
   B) Asian or Pacific Islander
   C) Black
   D) White
   E) Hispanic origin
   Answer: E

3. On most measures of socioeconomic status, Americans of Hispanic origin rank:
   A) higher than the general United States population.
   B) lower than the general United States population.
   C) about the same as the general United States population.
   Answer: B

4. It was not until relatively recently (late 1980s) that most states included a Hispanic-origin item on their:
   A) birth certificates.
   B) death certificates.
   C) driver's licenses.
   D) marriage license.
   Answer: B

5. Some health care officials feel the infant mortality rate is lower in two racial/ethinic groups because of the excellent social support provided by family members. In what two groups is this true?
   A) Americans of Hispanic origin and white Americans
   B) White Americans and Native Americans
   C) Americans of Hispanic origin and Native Americans
   D) Black Americans and Asian Americans
   Answer: C

6. The fastest growing minority group in the United States is:
   A) Native Americans.
   B) Asian/Pacific Islanders.
   C) black Americans.
   D) Americans of Hispanic origin.
   Answer: B

7. Greater respect for age, rank, status, and power are a part of the values of what minority group?
   A) Native Americans
   B) Asian/Pacific Islanders
   C) black Americans
   D) white Americans
   Answer: B

8. Which minority group has the lowest infant mortality rate?
   A) Native Americans
   B) Asian/Pacific Islanders
   C) black Americans
   D) Americans of Hispanic origin
   Answer: B

9. The resurgence of tuberculosis in the United States is linked to:
   A) poverty and substance abuse.
   B) substandard housing and homelessness.
   C) limited public health clinics.
   D) all the above
   E) just A and B
   Answer: D

10. Which minority group has the highest rate of years of potential life lost?
    A) Native Americans
    B) Asian/Pacific Islanders
    C) black Americans
    D) white Americans
    Answer: C

11. Inheritance of a sickle cell gene from only one parent will result in:
    A) sickle cell disease.
    B) sickle cell trait.
    C) sickle cell virus.
    D) sickle cell anemia.
    Answer: B

12. Almost a third of all hypertensives in the United States are:
    A) Native Americans.
    B) Asian/Pacific Islanders.
    C) black Americans.
    D) Americans of Hispanic origin.
    Answer: C

13. Which minority group has shown a great appreciation, respect and reverence for the land?
    A) Native Americans
    B) Asian/Pacific Islanders
    C) black Americans
    D) Americans of Hispanic origin
    Answer: A

14. Few Native Americans die of:
    A) cancer and stroke.
    B) suicide.
    C) homocide.
    D) motor vehicle crashes.
    Answer: A

15. The Indian Health Service was created in:
    A) 1876.
    B) 1901.
    C) 1925.
    D) 1954.
    Answer: D

16. There are three leading theories -historical, physiological, and social -for explaining what
    health problem?
    A) AIDS in Americans of Hispanic origin
    B) alcoholism in Native Americans
    C) Tuberculosis in Asian/Pacific Islanders
    D) violence in white Americans
    Answer. B

17. Those individuals who migrate to another country for the purpose of seeking permanent residence
    and hopefully a better life are referred to as:
    A) refugees.
    B) immigrants.
    C) aliens.
    D) illegal aliens.
    Answer: B

18. Which is the better predictor of health status?
    A) place of residence
    B) socioeconomic status
    C) gender
    D) racial/ethnic group
    Answer: B

19. _____ power brings with it access to "bases" of production such as
    information, knowledge and skills, participation in organization, and financial resources.
    A) Social
    B) Political
    C) Psychological
    D) Physiological
    Answer: A

20. For a group to be empowered, which of the "powers" must it first obtain?
    A) social
    B) political
    C) psychological
    D) physiological
    Answer: A

True-False

Write T if the statement is true and F if the statement is false.

1. In 1991, one American in seven spoke a language other than English at home.
   Answer: True

2. The number of interracial marriages in the United States was about 4 times greater in 1992 than in 1980.
   Answer: False

3. In its statistical reporting, the United States only recognizes two ethnic orgins.
   Answer: True

4. Epidemiological data have repeatedly shown that mortality rates of foreign-born and native-born within the same minority category are about the same.
   Answer: False

5. Hispanic origin is an ethnicity classification, not a race.
   Answer: True

6. Great sense of obligation to one's family, and accompanying feelings of shame and guilt if the obligations are ignored is a value of most Asian/Pacific Islanders.
   Answer: True

7. The reported number of tuberculosis cases in the United States today is greater than the cases reported in the early 1950s.
   Answer: False

8. Much of the disparity that exists today between the health care provided for black Americans compared to white Americans can be traced to slavery.
   Answer: True

9. Today many black Americans find it difficult to gain access to health care because of discrimination.
   Answer: True

10. Health status of black Americans has improved significantly in the last 40 years, but continues to lag behind other racial/ethnic subgroups.
    Answer: True

11. Black American infants die at a rate of about twice that of their white counterparts.
    Answer: True

12. Sickle cell disease is a genetic disease.
Answer: True

13. Sickle cell disease can be present in other racial groups besides blacks.
Answer: True

14. Central to Native American culture is that the people strive for a close integration within the family, clan and tribe and live in harmony with their environment.
Answer: True

15. Few Native Americans die from violent causes.
Answer: False

16. Tribal sovereignty is perhaps the most important Indian issue.
Answer: True

17. Aliens are people born in and owing allegiance to a country other than the one in which they live.
Answer: True

18. Few refugees currently entering the United States arrive from Third World countries.
Answer: False

19. Solutions to the community health problems of racial/ethnic minorities must be culturally sensitive.
Answer: True

20. Political power includes being able to vote, the power of voice, and collective action.
Answer: True

Essay

Write your answer in the space provided or on a separate sheet of paper.

1. What are the three primary reasons for the increase in minority groups in the United States?
Answer: (1) The birth and fertility rates of minorities living in this country are higher than those of the majority, (2) immigration into the United States continues, and (3) the number of interracial marriages is increasing.

2. Why is there such a disparity between the health status of black Americans compared to white Americans?
Answer: (1) Access to health care, (2) poverty, (3) less education, and (4) employment status.

3. Identify the two primary reasons why the infant mortality rate is so high in black Americans.
Answer: (1) Lack of family planning services, and (2) lack of prenatal care.

4. Briefly describe how the Indian Health Service fulfills its goal "to raise the health status of American Indians and Alaskan Natives to the highest possible level."
   Answer: (1) Assists Indian tribes in developing their health programs, (2) facilitates and assists Indian tribes in coordinating health resources, (3) provides comprehensive health care services, and (4) serves as the principal Federal advocate for Indians in the health field.

5. Identify some of the problems that have surfaced for many of the new refugees in the United States.
   Answer: (1) Lack of jobs, (2) lack of housing to fit socioeconomic levels, (3) lack of access to health care, (4) cultural barriers, and (5) backlash movements against refugees.

6. What steps could be taken to solve many of the community health problems of the racial and ethnic groups?
   Answer: (1) Change socioeconomic status, (2) provide universal access to health services, and (3) empower self and community.

Matching

Choose the item from Column 2 that best matches each item in Column 1.

Match the following descriptions with the appropriate racial/ethnic groups.

1. slow in being recognized on death certificates   Americans of Hispanic origin

2. the single largest minority   black Americans

3. highest rate of YPLL   black Americans

4. has a specific public health agency to raise the health of the population   Native Americans

5. very favorable health status   Asian/Pacific Islanders

6. Tuberculosis disproportionally affects this group.   Asian/Pacific Islanders

7. highest proportion of population living in poverty   Black Americans

8. hard hit by AIDS/HIV   Americans of Hispanic origin and Black Americans

9. highest infant mortality rate   Black Americans

10. fastest growing minority group in the United States   Asian/Pacific Islanders

11. cultural barriers   refugees

12. Sickle cell disease   Black Americans

13. backlash movement   refugees

14. alcohol problem   Native Americans

Chapter 10   Seniors

Multiple-Choice

Choose the one alternative that best completes the statement or answers the question.

1. Those individuals who are 75 years of age and older have been referred to as:
   A) old.
   B) young old.
   C) old old.
   D) oldest old.
   Answer: C

2. The study of aging from the broadest perspective is known as:
   A) ageism.
   B) gerontology.
   C) geriatrics.
   D) agology.
   Answer: B

3. From social and legislative standpoints, people in the United States are considered old when they reach the age of:
   A) 85.
   B) 75.
   C) 65.
   D) 55.
   Answer: C

4. The base of the traditional age-pyramid represents:
   A) the oldest and fewest number of people.
   B) high mortality.
   C) limited life expectancy.
   D) the youngest and largest number of people.
   Answer: D

5. The fastest growing age group in the United States is the:
   A) old.
   B) young old.
   C) old old.
   D) oldest old.
   Answer: D

6. The baby boomers include those individuals who were born between:
   A) 1926 and 1944.
   B) 1936 and 1954.
   C) 1946 and 1964.
   D) 1956 and 1974.
   Answer: C

7. The greatest immigration in the United States occurred between the:
    A) end of the Civil War and the beginning of the Great Depression.
    B) end of World War I and the beginning of the Great Depression.
    C) end of the Great Depression and the beginning of World War II.
    D) end of World War II and the beginning of the Vietnam War.
    Answer: A

8. _____ is a comparison between those individuals whom society
    considers economically productive and those it considers economically unproductive.
    A) Dependency ratio
    B) Youth dependency ratio
    C) Elderly dependency ratio.
    D) Labor-force ratio.
    Answer: D

9. The state with the greatest number of seniors living in it is:
    A) California.
    B) Florida.
    C) Texas.
    D) Arizona.
    Answer: A

10. Which of the following expenses usually increases for most seniors after retirement?
    A) mortgage payments
    B) health care
    C) professional association dues
    D) clothing
    Answer: B

11. Seniors depend most heavily on what source of income?
    A) public assistance
    B) earnings from jobs
    C) social security
    D) income from assets
    Answer: C

12. What percent of those age 65+ live in group housing?
    A) 6
    B) 16
    C) 26
    D) 36
    Answer: A

13. The single biggest housing need facing seniors is:
    A) finding a house in a nice location.
    B) locating housing in the suburbs.
    C) finding housing that is large enough for their needs.
    D) availability of affordable housing.
    Answer: D

14. According to Atchley, which of the following would not be included in the ideal solution to the transportation needs of seniors?
A) Fare reductions or discounts for all public transportation.
B) Subsidies to insure adequate scheduling and routing of present public transportation.
C) Subsidized taxi fares for the disabled and infirmed.
D) Building of mass transit systems in all major metropolitan areas.
E) Funds for senior centers to purchase and equip vehicles to transport seniors properly.
Answer: D

15. The services and facilities available to seniors was greatly enhanced by which amendments to the Older Americans Act of 1965?
A) National Nutritional Program for Seniors
B) Area Agencies on Aging
C) Title II
D) Title IV
Answer: B

16. The availability of these services allows many seniors to live semi-independently and delays their moving in with relatives or into group housing.
A) meal service
B) homemaker service
C) adult day care
D) respite care service
Answer: B

17. Which of the following is (are) problems faced by caregivers?
A) decreased personal freedom
B) lack of privacy
C) constant demands on their time and energy
D) all the above
E) just A and B
Answer: D

True-False

Write T if the statement is true and F if the statement is false.

1. Age is and always will be relative.
Answer: True

2. Since 1950, both the number of elderly and the proportion in the total United States population have grown significantly.
Answer: True

3. The United States is one of the few countries in the world where the elderly population is growing.
Answer: False

4. Since the end of the baby boom years, the fertility rate in the United States has steadily increased.
   Answer: False

5. In the United States, the life expectancy of all men and all blacks have always trailed women and whites, respectively.
   Answer: True

6. Historically, in the United States, net migration has resulted in population gain; more people immigrate than emigrate.
   Answer: True

7. Currently, the youth dependency ratio is greater than the elderly dependency ratio.
   Answer: True

8. The ratio of workers to dependents will be greater in the future than it is today.
   Answer: True

9. Most senior women remain married until they die.
   Answer: False

10. Men who lose a spouse through death or divorce are more likely to remarry than women in the same situation.
    Answer: True

11. The majority of noninstitutionalized seniors live with someone else (spouse, relative or friend).
    Answer: True

12. Since most seniors do not work, they are economically more vulnerable to circumstances beyond their control.
    Answer: True

13. Probably the single biggest change in housing needs of seniors is the need for special modifications because of physical disabilities.
    Answer: True

14. Continuing-care retirement communities (CCRCs) are a housing alternative for the well-to-do seniors as well as the poor seniors.

    Answer: True

16. Medicare has a primary role of financing acute health care services.
    Answer: True

17. Transportation is of prime importance to seniors because it enables them to remain independent.
    Answer: True

18. Activities of Daily Living (ADLs) can be used to measure functional limitations.
Answer: True

19. An informal caregiver can be a care-provider, but not a care-manager.
Answer: False

20. The need for personal care for seniors is projected to decrease in the coming years.
Answer: False

Essay

Write your answer in the space provided or on a separate sheet of paper.

1. List at least five myths of aging, then explain why each is a myth.
Answer: (1) After age 65, life goes steadily downhill. There is no magic age that defines such a point. (2) Old people are all alike. Seniors have many differences. (3) Old people are lonely and ignored by their families. Most seniors are regularly in contact with their families. (4) Old people are senile. Only about 5% are senile. (5) Old people have a good life. Most seniors still face many concerns. (6) Most old people are sickly. Most live active lifestyles. (7) Old people no longer have any sexual interest or ability. Sexual interest does not diminish with age. (8) Most old peo

2. Draw and label the traditional age-pyramid.
Answer: picture of triangle; starting from the bottom going up -youngest and largest number of people, the middle -sloping sides indicate high mortality and limited life expectancy, and at the top -oldest and fewest people.

3. What are the three factors that affect the size and age of a population.
Answer: (1) fertility rates, (2) mortality rates, and (3) the migration of individuals from one country to another

4. Explain the difference between dependency ratio and labor-force dependency ratio.
Answer: Labor-force dependency ratios differ from dependency ratios in that they are based on the number of people who are actually working and those who are not, independent of their ages.

5. What are the five essential needs that determine lifestyles of people of all ages?
Answer: (1) income, (2) housing, (3) health care, (4) transportation, and (5) community facilities and services

6. With regard to transportation, what three categories can be used to classify seniors?
Answer: (1) those who can use the present forms of transportation whether it be their own vehicle or public transportation (2) those who could use public transportation if the barriers of cost and access were removed (3) those who need special services beyond those available through public transportation

Matching

Choose the item from Column 2 that best matches each item in Column 1.

Match the following descriptions with the appropriate age group.

1. young old   65 to 74 years old

2. oldest old   85 years of age and older

3. elderly   60 years of age and older

4. old old   75 to 84 years old

5. age for Social Security   65 years of age

Match the following activities with the appropriate service.

6. yard work   chore and home maintenance service

7. social contacts   visitor service

8. modeled after child day care   adult day care service

9. Meals-on-Wheels   meal service

10. possible site for congregate meals   senior centers

11. may be paid for by Medicare   home health care service

12. house cleaning   homemaker service

13. plumbing and electrical repairs   chore and home maintenance service

14. requested by informal caregivers respite care service

15. congregate meals   meal service

Chapter 11   Community Mental Health

Multiple-Choice

Choose the one alternative that best completes the statement or answers the question.

1. Adults with good mental health are able to:
    A) function under difficulty, show considerations for others.
    B) love others, curb hate and guilt.
    C) maintain control over their tension and anxiety.
    D) all the above
    E) just A and C
    Answer: D

2. Which of the following is (are) causes of mental disorders?
    A) mental deficiency at birth
    B) physical (or physiological) impairment
    C) psychological causes
    D) all the above
    Answer: D

3. Deinstitutionalization of mental health patients began in which decade?
    A) 1940s
    B) 1950s
    C) 1960s
    D) 1970s
    Answer: B

4. Which of the following statements about chlorpromazine is not true?
    A) Referred to as a chemical straight jacket.
    B) It is an antipsychotic drug.
    C) The most widely used of the initial mental disorder drugs.
    D) It was outlawed by the FDA in 1954.
    Answer: D

5. The Mental Retardation Facilities and Community Mental Health Centers (CMHC) Act was passed during the presidency of:
    A) Franklin Pierce.
    B) John Kennedy.
    C) Jimmy Carter.
    D) George Bush.
    Answer: B

6. Which center of SAMHSA is working to respond to the growing crisis of mental, emotional, and behavior problems among the youth?
    A) Center for Substance Abuse Treatment
    B) Center for Substance Abuse Prevention
    C) Center for Mental Health Services
    Answer: C

7. The General Accounting Office has estimated the proportion of homeless that are mentally ill to be at least:
   A) three-fourths.
   B) one-half.
   C) one-third.
   D) one-tenth.
   Answer: C

8. Which of the following is (are) true about the homeless?
   A) Approximately one-third are mentally ill.
   B) The incidence of tuberculosis is higher in the homeless than the domiciled persons.
   C) Trauma occurs at a rate 2 - 3 times higher among homeless than among domiciled persons.
   D) all the above are true
   E) just A and B are true
   Answer: D

9. _____ involves treatment of the mentally ill with medications.
   A) Biomedical therapy
   B) Psychotherapy
   C) Behavioral therapy
   Answer: A

10. Biofeedback, stress management and relaxation training are forms of what type of therapy to treat mental illness?
    A) biomedical therapy
    B) psychotherapy
    C) behavioral therapy
    Answer: C

11. In what year was the Substance Abuse and Mental Health Services Administration (SAMHSA) established?
    A) 1952
    B) 1962
    C) 1982
    D) 1992
    Answer: D

12. Which of the following are required services of community mental health centers?
    A) inpatient and partial hospitalization
    B) outpatient and emergency care
    C) consultation and education services
    D) all the above
    E) just B and C
    Answer: D

13. Which of the following is not true about the platform of the National Alliance for the Mentally Ill?
    A) Expediting of the development of neuroleptic drugs.
    B) Eradication of family therapy.
    C) Return of NIMH into the NIH.
    D) Mental disorders are caused by the environment.
    Answer: D

True-False

Write T if the statement is true and F if the statement is false.

1. It has been estimated that as many as three in five persons will need hospitalization for mental illness in their lifetime.
   Answer: False

2. Adults who have good mental health are able to find more satisfaction in giving than receiving.
   Answer: True

3. Adults who have good mental health are able to change or adapt to changes about them.
   Answer: True

4. The most often cited reference for the classification of mental disorders is the Diagnostic and Statistical Manual of Mental Disorders (Third Edition - Revised).
   Answer: True

5. Suicide and homicide are social indicators of mental illness.
   Answer: True

6. Individuals under stress consume less alcohol, smoke more cigarettes, and drink more coffee than those under less stress.
   Answer: False

7. "Social Darwinism" was often used to justify the removal of misfits and mad persons to state run institutions where they could receive custodial care.
   Answer: True

8. As a result of World War II, new crisis intervention methods were developed and the image of psychiatry was improved.
   Answer: True

9. During World War II, it was not uncommon for conscientious objectors to spend their war years working in mental institutions.
   Answer: True

10. About three-fourths of the United States population is now served by a community mental health center (CMHC).
    Answer: False

11. Finally, in 1990, it could be stated that the United States had a national mental health program.
    Answer: False

12. The large number of mentally ill homeless in the United States in the 1990s is considered a legacy of deinstitutionalization.
    Answer: True

13. The incidence of tuberculosis is higher in the homeless.
    Answer: True

14. The task of providing primary mental health services falls mainly on the private, voluntary agencies, such as the National Mental Health Association and its affiliates.
    Answer: True

15. Electroconvulsive treatment (ECT) for mental illness is a form of psychotherapy.
    Answer: False

16. Psychotherapy is most likely to be successful in less severe cases of emotional distress.
    Answer: True

17. In involuntary outpatient commitment, both patient and provider alike are coerced into maintaining scheduled treatment for the good of all.
    Answer: True

Essay

Write your answer in the space provided or on a separate sheet of paper.

1. Briefly describe the characteristics of people with good mental health.
   Answer: People with good mental health possess a good self image, feel right about other people, and are able to meet the demands of every day life.

2. What was included in the mental health therapy known as moral treatment?
   Answer: Mentally ill people were removed from the everyday life stresses and given asylum in a quiet country environment. They received a regimen of rest, light food, exercise, fresh air, and amusements. They were cared for by a caring and respectful staff.

3. What were the four forces that propelled deinstitutionalization of mental health patients in the United States.
   Answer: (1) economics, (2) idealism, (3) legal considerations, and (4) the development and marketing of antipsychotic drugs

4. Why did Medicare and Medicaid add greatly to the care of the mentally ill?
   Answer: Medicare provided hospital and physician services for the aged and Medicaid provided grants to the states for medical assistance to indigent persons. A remarkable feature of these amendments was the inclusion of psychiatric benefits.

5. Why were the 1980s, the "me decade," bad for mental health care?
    Answer: Federal spending for many health and social programs was reduced. These cuts had a great impact on the deinstitutionalized, chronically, mentally ill people.

6. What are the major mental health problems faced by the United States in the 1990s?
    Answer: (1) large number of homeless mentally ill, (2) the continued lack of a comprehensive, coordinated system of services for the mentally ill in most communities, (3) the absence of national leadership in setting a mental health policy, and (4) the need for better treatments

7. What is meant by the statement that "the 1990s is the decade of the brain"?
    Answer: There is great anticipation that during the 1990s research on the brain will yield significant new knowledge about how the brain works and will bring with it significant breakthroughs in the treatment of mental disorders.

Matching

Choose the item from Column 2 that best matches each item in Column 1.

Match the following descriptions with the appropriate "stress" term.

1.	third stage of general adaptation syndrome	stage of exhaustion
2.	body tries to adapt to stressor	stage of resistance
3.	ulcers	disease of adaptation
4.	body prepares to resist stressor	alarm reaction
5.	marriage	stressor
6.	includes fight or flight reaction	alarm reaction
7.	could include physical disease and death	stage of exhaustion
8.	divorce	stressor
9.	being stuck in traffic	stressor
10.	high blood pressure	disease of adaptation

Match the following activity with the person who is associated with the activity.

11.	built the Pennsylvania Hospital	Thomas Bond
12.	lobbied for the state to care for the mentally ill	Dorothea Dix

13. active in the mental hygiene movement   Adolf Meyer

14. began the therapy known as moral   William Tuke
    treatment

15. founded the National Committee on   Clifford W. Beers
    Mental Hygiene that later became the
    National Mental Health Association.

Match the following mental health activity with its related time period or event.

16. first attempt at attacking mental   mental hygiene movement
    health problem at the community level

17. movement of mentally ill to quiet,   moral mental health treatment era
    country environment

18. era during which antipsychotic drugs   deinstitutionalization
    were developed and marketed

19. mental health care was gruesome   nineteenth Century

20. movement to institutionalize the   state hospitals
    mentally ill

21. establishment of National Institute of   after World War II
    Mental Health (NIMH)

22. created by then president John F.   Community Mental Health Centers (CMHC)
    Kennedy

23. time when mental illness was recognized   community support movement
    as a social welfare problem

Chapter 12   Abuse of Alcohol and Other Drugs

Multiple-Choice

Choose the one alternative that best completes the statement or answers the question.

1. According to the 1992 survey on drug use, abuse of illicit drugs among young Americans in high school and college has:
   A) continued to decline since 1979.
   B) continued to increase since 1979.
   C) stayed about the same since 1979.
   Answer: A

2. According to the 1992 survey on drug use, the number one illicit drug used by high school seniors and college students is:
   A) cocaine.
   B) marijuana.
   C) tobacco.
   D) crack cocaine.
   Answer: B

3. The most serious drug problem in the United States is:
   A) marijuana.
   B) cocaine.
   C) alcohol.
   D) tobacco.
   Answer: C

4. Which of the following best describes "when one discontinues the use of a prescribed antibiotic before the entire prescribed dose is completed or, when one takes four aspirin rather than two aspirin as specified on the label"?
   A) drug use
   B) drug abuse
   C) drug misuse
   D) drug dependence
   Answer: C

5. _____ is a non-valuative term referring to drug taking behavior in general, regardless of whether the behavior is appropriate.
   A) Drug use
   B) Drug abuse
   C) Drug misuse
   D) Drug dependence
   Answer: A

6. What do alcohol, nicotine, non-prescription and prescription drugs have in common?
   A) They are all illicit drugs.
   B) They are all legal drugs.
   C) They are all illegal drugs.
   D) They are all inexpensive.
   Answer: B

7. Tobacco use increases one's risk for all the following except:
   A) heart disease.
   B) stress.
   C) lung cancer.
   D) stroke.
   Answer: B

8. Environmental tobacco smoke has been causally associated with:
   A) lung cancer.
   B) new cases of asthma in children.
   C) lower respiratory infections in children.
   D) all the above.
   E) none of the above.
   Answer: D

9. _____ are substances that have a high potential for abuse, have no accepted medical uses and no acceptable standards for safe use.
   A) Designer drugs
   B) Hallucinogens
   C) Dangerous drugs
   Answer: C

10. Designer drugs get their name because they are:
    A) made for a specific group of people.
    B) designed to mimic popular psychoactive compounds.
    C) very expensive.
    Answer: B

11. Testosterone and human growth hormone are considered what kind of drugs?
    A) depressents
    B) anabolic drugs
    C) hallucinogens
    D) stimulants
    Answer: B

12. Which group of drugs are useful in the rebuilding of muscles after starvation or disease and for the treatment of dwarfism?
    A) stimulants
    B) depressants
    C) anabolic drugs
    D) narcotics
    Answer: C

13. All of the following are side effects found in men who use anabolic drugs except:
    A) acne.
    B) gynecomastia (development of breasts).
    C) reduction in testicular size.
    D) increased body hair.
    Answer: D

14. Which of the following is often a drug of choice of the young because of availability and low cost?
    A) depressants
    B) inhalants
    C) designer drugs
    D) anabolic drugs
    Answer: B

15. Increasing the price of alcohol or increasing cigarette taxes are examples of what level of drug abuse prevention?
    A) primary
    B) secondary
    C) tertiary
    D) none of the above
    Answer: A

16. Which of the following best describes the federal governments approach to drug abuse prevention?
    A) Heavy funding to reduce the supply.
    B) Heavy funding to reduce demand.
    C) Equal funding for supply and demand.
    Answer: A

17. Of the federal level departments involved in drug control, which one has the largest budget to fight drug abuse?
    A) Department of Justice
    B) Department of the Treasury
    C) Department of Health and Human Services
    D) Department of Defense
    Answer: A

18. Which of the following Department of Justice agencies is responsible for investigating and assisting in the prosecution of drug traffickers and their accomplices in the United States and abroad,and seizes the drugs as well as the assets on which they depend?
    A) Federal Bureau of Investigation
    B) Drug Enforcement Agency
    C) Immigration and Naturalization Services
    D) Organized Crime Drug Enforcement Task Force
    Answer: B

19. Which of the following agencies within the DHHS is primarily involved in drug abuse research?
    A) Substance Abuse and Mental Health Services Administration
    B) The Center for Substance Abuse Prevention
    C) National Institute of Drug Abuse
    D) Food and Drug Administration
    Answer: C

20. At the local level in the Governor's Commission for a Drug Free Indiana, emphasis is placed on:
    A) education and law enforcement.
    B) intervention and treatment.
    C) supply and education.
    D) just A and B
    E) just B and C
    Answer: D

21. In the Drug Abuse Resistance Education (DARE) program, what groups of people present the lessons in the elementary school classroom?
    A) elementary classroom teachers
    B) police officers
    C) health educators
    D) school nurses
    Answer: B

True-False

Write T if the statement is true and F if the statement is false.

1. The abuse of alcohol and other drugs is one of America's most expensive community health problems.
   Answer: True

2. Pyschoactive drugs are drugs that affect the central nervous system.
   Answer: True

3. The most serious drug problem in the United States is marijuana.
   Answer: False

4. Because illicit drugs have no approved medical uses, any illicit drug use is considered drug abuse.
   Answer: True

5. It is possible to be both psychologically and physically dependent to a drug at the same time.
   Answer: True

6. Type II inherited alcoholism is also known as milieu limited.
   Answer: False

7. Alochol has been found to increase one's risk of involvement in both intentional and unintentional injuries.
   Answer: True

8. Nicotine is the psychoactive and addictive drug present in tobacco products.
Answer: True

9. Environmental tobacco smoke (ETS) has been casually linked to lung cancer deaths.
Answer: True

10. Most over-the-counter drugs have the ability to provide consumers with a cure for their problems.
Answer: False

11. One serious consequence of the misuse of prescription drugs is the development of drug resistant strains of pathogens.
Answer: True

12. Hallucinogens cause a phenomenon known as synesthesia.
Answer: True

13. Anabolic drugs do have legitimate medical uses.
Answer: True

14. There are only two cabinet level departments in the federal government that are involved in drug control and receive funds to reduce alcohol and other drug problems.
Answer: False

15. The Department of Justice addresses the demand side of the drug trade.
Answer: False

10. The Department of Health and Human Services address the demand side of the drug trade.
Answer: True

17. The Food and Drug Administration is more concerned with drug misuse than abuse.
Answer: True

18. Student Assistance Programs (SAPs) are school based programs modeled after employee assistance programs in the workplace.
Answer: True

19. Small companies are more likely than large companies to have the major components of a drug-free workplace program.
Answer: False

Essay

Write your answer in the space provided or on a separate sheet of paper.

1. Why do abusers of alcohol and other drugs represent a serious threat to the community?
Answer: (1) They have greater health care needs, (2) suffer more injuries, and (3) are less productive than those who do not.

2. Identify the four major environmental risk factors that contribute to substance abuse and give an example of each.

Answer: (a) personal factors -impulsiveness, depressive mood, stress, personality disturbances; (b) home and family life -family structure, family dynamics, family problems, negative family events, family attitudes toward alcohol and drug use; (c) school and peer groups -perceived and actual drug use by peers; (d) sociocultural environment -social ecology, one's neighborhood

3. Alcohol reinforces the user in what two ways?

Answer: (1) it lowers anxieties, and (2) produces a mild euphoria

4. Name the three levels of drug abuse prevention and give an example of each.

Answer: A. Primary -raising price of alcohol or tobacco, arresting a drug pusher B. Secondary -programs aimed at drug users C. Tertiary -programs designed to provide treatment for abuse and aftercare, including relapse prevention

5. How do two agencies in the Department of Treasury -the United States Customs Service and the Internal Revenue Service -get involved in the control of the drug problem?

Answer: The United States Customs Service works with the DEA to target the transportation of drugs and to intercept drugs crossing our borders. The IRS targets major traffickers by investigating money laundering operations and prosecuting tax evasion cases.

6. Identify the six key features for a successful community-based drug education program.

Answer: (1) a comprehensive strategy; (2) an indirect approach to drug abuse prevention; (3) the goal of empowering youth; (4) a participatory approach; (5) a culturally sensitive orientation; (6) highly structured activities.

7. List the five facets of a typical workplace substance abuse program.

Answer: (1) formal written substance abuse policy that reflects the employer's committment to a drug-free workplace; (2) employee drug education and awareness program; (3) supervisor training program; (4) employee assistance program; (5) drug testing program.

8. What do these organizations have in common -Mothers Against Drunk Driving, Students Against Drunk Driving, Alcoholics Anonymous, and Narcotics Anonymous?

Answer: unofficial agencies founded to prevent or control the social and personal consequences of drug and alcohol abuse

Matching

Choose the item from Column 2 that best matches each item in Column 1.

Match the following descriptions with the appropriate substance.

1. aspirin   over-the-counter

2. used to self-medicate   over-the-counter drug

3. Valium   prescription drug

4. number one drug problem in the United States

    alcohol

5. found in tobacco

    nicotine

6. contributing factor to 40% of all crashes with occupant deaths

    alcohol

7. mouth washes

    over-the-counter drug

8. purchased only with a physican's or dentist's written instructions

    prescription drug

9. marijuana

    illegal drug

10. opium, morphine, heroin

    narcotics

Match the following substances with the appropriate origin.

11. marijuana

    comes from the hemp plant

12. cocaine

    comes from the coca plant

13. opium

    comes from the poppy plant

14. morphine

    comes from the poppy plant

15. hash oil

    comes from the hemp plant

16. heroin

    comes from the poppy plant

17. hashish

    comes from the hemp plant

18. cat

    comes from the khat plant

Match the following descriptions with the classification of drugs.

19. cocaine

    stimulant(s)

20. slows down the nervous system

    depressant(s)

21. protein building drugs

    anabolic drug(s)

22. LSD

    hallucinogen(s)

23. amphetamines

    stimulant(s)

24. paint solvents and cosmetics

    inhalants

25. speed up the nervous system

    stimulant(s)

26. alcohol   depressant(s)

27. can cause bad trips   hallucinogen(s)

28. china white (alpha methyl fentanyl)   designer drug(s)

29. often misused by athletes   anabolic drug(s)

30. breathable chemicals   inhalants

Multiple-Choice

Choose the one alternative that best completes the statement or answers the question.

1. Before _____ most health care in the United States took place in the patient's home.
   A) 1940
   B) 1920
   C) 1900
   D) 1850
   Answer: D

2. During the latter portion of which century did the scientific method begin to play a more important role in health care?
   A) twentieth
   B) nineteenth
   C) eighteenth
   D) seventeenth
   Answer: B

3. The leading causes of death at the beginning of the twentieth century were:
   A) noncommunicable diseases.
   B) noninfectious diseases.
   C) communicable disease.
   D) adult onset diseases.
   Answer: C

4. The primary reason for the passage of the Hill-Burton Act in 1946 was to:
   A) provide substantial funds for hospital construction.
   B) provide money to purchase medicine for underserved areas.
   C) create a health care system for WWII veterans.
   D) provide funds to remodel old hospitals.
   Answer: A

5. In the third party payment system for health care, the third party is the:
   A) patient.
   B) health care provider.
   C) insurance company.
   D) hospital.
   Answer: C

6. In the third party payment system for health care, the second party is:
   A) patient.
   B) health care provider.
   C) insurance company.
   D) hospital.
   Answer: B

7. In the third party payment system for health care, the first party is the:
   A) patient.
   B) health care provider.
   C) insurance company.
   D) hospital.
   Answer: A

8. Which type of care is provided in nursing homes, facilities for the mentally and emotionally disturbed, adult and senior day care centers and in the home?
   A) primary health care
   B) secondary health care
   C) tertiary health care
   D) continuing health care
   Answer: D

9. The greatest need for health care workers will continue to be in:
   A) rural areas.
   B) inner-city areas.
   C) suburban areas.
   D) all the above.
   E) just A and B.
   Answer: E

10. Early educational training for this health care provider group was based on manipulating the musculoskeletal system.
    A) allopathic providers
    B) osteopathic providers
    C) nonallopathic
    D) none of the above
    Answer: B

11. Those physicians who decide to specialize in a particular field of medicine must complete a (an):
    A) residency.
    B) internship.
    C) practicum.
    D) field experience.
    Answer: A

12. Registered nurses holding a bachelor of science in nursing degree are referred to as:
    A) technical nurses.
    B) prodical nurses.
    C) professional nurses.
    D) vocational nurses.
    Answer: C

13. These professionals assist, facilitate and complement the work of physicians and other health care specialists.
    A) osteopathic providers
    B) allied health care professionals
    C) limited care providers
    D) allopathic providers
    Answer: B

14. Public health clinics are primary funded by:
    A) donations.
    B) tax dollars.
    C) insurance payments.
    D) fees for service.
    Answer: B

15. Non-profit hospitals are referred to as:
    A) private hospitals.
    B) voluntary hospitals.
    C) governmental hospitals.
    D) full service hospitals.
    Answer: B

16. Those providers who would commonly work in a rehabilitation center include:
    A) physical therapists.
    B) occupational therapists.
    C) respiratory therapists.
    D) all the above
    E) just A and B
    Answer: D

True-False

Write T if the statement is true and F if the statement is false.

1. At best, health care in the United States is delivered by providers who are linked by informal communication.
   Answer: True

2. War time has traditionally been a time when many new applications in medicine have been discovered.
   Answer: True

3. The debate over whether health care was a basic right or priviledge in America began in the late 1960s.
   Answer: False

4. The third party payment system for health care became solidified as the standard method of payment for health care costs in the 1940s.
   Answer: False

5. Medicare and Medicaid were enacted in 1965 to increase citizen access to health care.
   Answer: True

6. The purpose of the Health System Agencies that were developed in the mid-1970s was to cut costs by preventing the building of "unnecessary" facilities or the purchase of unnecessary equipment.
   Answer: True

7. Home health care is that care that is provided in personal residences.
   Answer: True

8. Approximately a third of all health care workers are employed in hospitals.
   Answer: False

9. Many insurance companies and Medicare and Medicaid provide reimbursement for chiropractic care.
   Answer: True

10. The present trend is to phase out licensed practical nurse/licensed vocational nurse training programs.
    Answer: True

11. A big difference between clinics and hospitals is that clinics do not have in-patient beds and hospitals do.
    Answer: True

12. Public health clinics are primarly funded by fees for the service provided.
    Answer: False

13. Recent growth in continuing care came about as a result of the current trend to discharge patients from hospitals earlier in their recovery to reduce health care costs.
    Answer: True

Essay

Write your answer in the space provided or on a separate sheet of paper.

1. Does the United States have a true health care system?
   Answer: Probably not. It provides medical treatment, not care; it is not a system but rather a haphazard conglomeration of medical entrepreneurs, and it focuses on disease not health.

2. List and briefly describe the six levels of care in the spectrum of health care delivery.
   Answer: (1) preventive care -refers to care provided to healthy individuals to keep them healthy; (2) primary care -front line or first contact care; (3) secondary care -involves intense and elaborate diagnosis and treatment; (4) tertiary (special) care -is advanced care that often requires highly technical services for patients; (5) resortative health care -provided after surgery, or other successful treatment, during remission in cases of an oncogenic disease, or when the progression of an incurable disease has been arrested; (6) continuing care -includes long-term care, care for chronic proble

3. Explain the chiropractors basic approach to treatment.
   Answer: (1) the identification of the misalignment through x-rays, and (2) the realignment of the bones through a series of treatments called "adjustments"

4. Explain the difference between a full service hospital and a limited service hospital.
   Answer: A full service hospital is one that offers care at all or most of the six levels of care while a limited service hospital offers only the specific services needed by the population served.

Matching

Choose the item from Column 2 that best matches each item in Column 1.

Match the following descriptions with the appropriate date.

1. third party payment system solidified | 1960s

2. health care bill reached 14% of the GNP | 1990s

3. communicable diseases leading cause of death | early 1900s

4. health care deregulation | 1980s

5. Medicare and Medicaid began | 1965

6. Hill Burton Act | 1946

7. health system agencies | 1974

Match the following descriptions with the type of care.

8. first contact care | primary heath care

9. advanced care, often requires highly technical services | tertiary health care

10. includes long-term care | continuing health care

11. given to healthy people to keep them healthy | preventive health care

12. provided after surgery or other successful treatment | restorative health care

13. involves intense and elaborate diagnosis and treatment | secondary health care

Match the following providers of health care with the appropriate descriptions.

14. chiropractors   nonallopathic

15. dentist   limited care provider

16. respiratory therapists   allied health care professionals

17. Doctors of Medicine (MDs)   allopathic provider

18. podiatrist   limited care provider

19. naturopaths   nonallopathic

20. nuclear medicine technicians   allied health care professionals

21. acupuncturists   nonallopathic

22. psychologist   limited care provider

23. Doctors of Osteopathic Medicine (DOs)   osteopathic provider

Chapter 14   Health Care System: Function

Multiple-Choice

Choose the one alternative that best completes the statement or answers the question.

1. The health care that is most difficult to obtain for those in the United States without access to care is:
    A) primary care.
    B) secondary care.
    C) tertiary care.
    D) emergency care.
    Answer: A

2. The primary factors that limit the access to health care in the United States are:
    A) health insurance and inadequate insurance.
    B) poverty.
    C) lack of physicians and hospitals.
    D) just A and B
    E) just B and C
    Answer: D

3. Those medically indigent who are working full time at low paying jobs that provide no health care benefits are referred to as:
    A) no access people.
    B) Medicaid recipients.
    C) the down and out.
    D) the working poor.
    Answer: D

4. The largest single expenditure faced by the United States each year is:
    A) defense.
    B) housing.
    C) health care.
    D) education.
    Answer: C

5. Approximately what percent of the United States health care bill is paid for via third party payments?
    A) 80
    B) 60
    C) 40
    D) 20
    Answer: A

6. The maximum amount an insurer will pay for a certain service is referred to as:
   A) deductible.
   B) coinsurance.
   C) fixed indemnity.
   D) exclusion.
   Answer: C

7. Many times pre-existing conditions become _____ in health insurance policies.
   A) deductibles
   B) coinsurance
   C) fixed indemnities.
   D) exclusions.
   Answer: D

8. The portion of Medicare that covers hospital costs and is referred to a contributory program is Part:
   A) A.
   B) B.
   C) C.
   D) D.
   Answer: A

9. Which of the following is (are) problems(s) associated with Medicare and Medicaid?
   A) non acceptance and fraud
   B) deductibles too high
   C) based on DRGs
   D) too many exclusions
   E) Bond D
   Answer: A

10. The national average cost of one year of nursing home care ranges from:
    A) $10,000 to $15,000.
    B) $15,000 to $20,000.
    C) $25,000 to $40,000 or more.
    D) $50,000 to $75,000 or more.
    Answer: C

11. In which of the four models of HMOs do physicians provide service to only those enrolled in the HMO?
    A) staff model
    B) group model
    C) network model
    D) independent practice association model
    Answer: A

12. "Doc in Box" refers to:
    A) HMOs.
    B) ambulatory care centers.
    C) EPOs and PPOs.
    D) none of the above
    Answer: B

13. The comprehensive approach to health care delivery that encompasses planning, education, monitoring, coordinating and controlling quality, access, and cost considering the interests of patients, providers and payers is called:
    A) managed care.
    B) open competition.
    C) cost containment.
    D) managed competition.
    Answer: A

14. Which of the following is (are) a strength(s) of the Canadian health care system compared to the United States?
    A) All citizens have health insurance.
    B) Administrative costs are lower.
    C) Less expensive to run.
    D) Emphasis placed on prevention and primary care.
    E) all the above
    Answer: E

15. The new Oregon health care plan cuts health care costs by:
    A) modifying Medicare.
    B) reducing Medicaid fraud.
    C) enhancing the medigap plans to cover all.
    D) not using Medicaid dollars to pay for health care that may not improve health status of the population.
    Answer: D

True-False

Write T if the statement is true and F if the statement is false.

1. Those who are unable to receive primary medical care because they cannot afford it are referred to as medically indigent.
   Answer: True

2. Often the medically indigent have full time jobs that provide no health care benefits.
   Answer: True

3. Sweden spends more per capita annually on health care than any other nation in the world.
   Answer: False

4. The health care system in the United States is referred to as a fee-for-service system.
   Answer: True

5. An increase in either the risk of the insured or the health care coverage provided will result in an increase in the cost of a health insurance policy.
   Answer: True

6. At the present time, government health insurance plans are only available to select groups in the United States.
   Answer: True

7. Those health care providers willing to accept Medicare patients must agree to accept the Medicare-approved amount as payment in full.
   Answer: True

8. Eligibility for enrollment in Medicaid is determined by the federal government.
   Answer: False

9. Like Medicare, Medicaid is a contributory health insurance program.
   Answer: False

10. Catastrophe health coverage is a part of Medicare.
    Answer: False

11. Under federal law there is a national standarization of medigap policies.
    Answer: True

12. Medigap is a supplemental insurance program specifically designed for those on Medicaid.
    Answer: False

13. Most nursing home cost are paid by Medicare.
    Answer: False

14. The majority of Americans are impoverished within the first year of making long-term health care payments.
    Answer: True

15. Health maintenance organizations are considered fee-for-service units.
    Answer: False

16. An HMO does not make money on treating ill people but on keeping people healthy.
    Answer: True

17. A major objection to both HMOs and PPOs is that the patients cannot freely select their provider.
    Answer: True

18. Managed competition for health care delivery is an approach that has not been tried anywhere in the world.
    Answer: True

19. The health care system in Canada is considered a socialized system.
    Answer: False

20. The major complaint of the Canadian health care system has been the rationing of certain types of care requiring high technology equipment and speciality physicians.
    Answer: True

21. The Oregon health plan was developed to restructure its Medicare plan.
    Answer: False

Essay

Write your answer in the space provided or on a separate sheet of paper.

1. What is meant by the phrase fee-for-service-system?
   Answer: Under this type of health care system people select a provider, receive a service (care), and pay the bill (a fee).

2. What is meant by the statement that health insurance is a risk and cost spreading process?
   Answer: The cost of one person's injury or illness is shared by all in the group. Each person in the group has a different chance (or risk) of having a problem and needing health care. The concept of insurance has everyone in the group, no matter what their risk, helping to pay for the collective risk of the group. The risk of costly ill health is spread in a reasonably equitable fashion among all persons purchasing insurance, and everyone is protected from having to pay an unsurmountable bill for a catastrophic injury or illness.

3. Why is it that when most organizations become self-insured they can cut their health care costs?
   Answer· The organization acts the parameters of the policy; deductibles, coinsurance, fixed indemnities, and exclusions.

4. What are two major problems that plague both Medicare and Medicaid? Describe each.
   Answer: (1) Some physicians and hospitals do not accept Medicare or Medicaid patients because of the tedious and time consuming paperwork, lengthy delays in reimbursement, and insufficent reimbursement. (2) A few physicians and hospitals file Medicare and Medicaid paperwork for care or services not rendered or rendered incompletely. This is known as Medicare/Medicaid fraud.

5. How have medigap policies been standardized by federal laws?
   Answer: (1) companies can offer no more than 10 plans; (2) each plan must have a core set of benefits; (3) plans are identified by letters A through J; (4) if a company sells medigap policies, it must offer plan A

6. How do preferred provider organizations and exclusive provider organizations differ?
   Answer: EPOs have stronger financial incentives to use a single provider.

7. How do preferred provider organizations and exclusive providers organizations cut health care costs?
   Answer: The organizations contract with providers to offer services to organization enrollees at a fixed (discount) rate.

8. What are the six major points of the American Health Security Act of 1993?
   Answer: (1) security; (2) cost control; (3) enhancing quality; (4) expanding access to care;
   (5) reducing bureaucracy; (6) reduce fraud and abuse

9. What four items must each provincial and territorial authority in Canada ensure about its
   health care plan?
   Answer: (1) All residents have access to care regardless of cost; (2) necessary hospital and
   physician services are available; (3) residents have continuous coverage as they
   travel from one province to another; and (4) the provincial programs are run as
   non-profit organizations.

Matching

Choose the item from Column 2 that best matches each item in Column 1.

Match the following descriptions with the appropriate insurance term.

1.	periodic payments by insurees	premiums
2.	obligations of the beneficiary	deductible and coinsurance
3.	health problem not covered by a policy	exclusion
4.	maximum amount an insurer will pay for a certain service	fixed indemnity
5.	a health problem of a new enrollee in a health insurance plan	pre-existing condition
6.	also known as a co-payment	coinsurance

Match the following descriptions with the appropriate type of health insurance.

7.	covers people 65 years of age and older	Medicare
8.	eligibility determined by each state	Medicaid
9.	covers people with permanent kidney failure	Medicare
10.	covers people on other types of welfare	Medicaid
11.	covers certain disabled people under age 65	Medicare
12.	uses a prospective pricing system	Medicare
13.	reimburses hospitals based upon DRGs	Medicare
14.	helps cover out-of-pocket expenses	medigap

15. policies defined by letters A through J   medigap

Match the following descriptions with the appropriate insurance term.

16. must be paid by the beneficiary before   deductible
the insurance company will pay

Chapter 15 Environmental Concerns: Wastes and Pollution

Multiple-Choice

Choose the one alternative that best completes the statement or answers the question.

1. Disease-producing agents would be considered what type of environmental hazard?
   A) biological
   B) chemical
   C) physical
   D) psychological
   Answer: A

2. Which of the following sources creates the greatest amount of solid waste?
   A) municipalities
   B) industry
   C) mining
   D) agriculture
   Answer: D

3. Municipal waste makes up what percent of the total solid waste in the United States?
   A) 5
   B) 10
   C) 25
   D) 50
   Answer: A

4. The major component of municipal waste is:
   A) food.
   B) yard waste.
   C) paper and paper products.
   D) wood and plastic.
   Answer: C

5. Which of the following statements is true with regards to handling solid waste?
   A) An equal amount of money is spent on collection and disposal.
   B) More money is spent on collection than disposal.
   C) More money is spent on disposal than collection.
   Answer: B

6. The components of an integrated waste-management approach include:
   A) sanitary landfills.
   B) recycling and source reduction.
   C) incineration.
   D) all the above
   E) just A and B
   Answer: D

7. Most municipal waste in the United States is disposed of via:
   A) sanitary landfills.
   B) incineration.
   C) recycling.
   Answer: A

8. Which of the following is (are) a benefit(s) of recycling?
   A) conserves resources
   B) conserves energy
   C) conserves sanitary landfill space
   D) all the above
   E) just A and C
   Answer: D

9. Which of the following statements about recycling is not true?
   A) The greatest recycling efforts in the United States took place during WWII.
   B) Japan recycles much more than the United States.
   C) The United States is no longer considered a throw-a-way society.
   D) Recycling can conserve energy, resources and landfill space.
   Answer: C

10. When the EPA tests a substance to determine if it is hazardous which of the following characteristics is not considered?
    A) corrosiveness
    B) ignitability
    C) toxicity
    D) biodegradable factors
    E) reactivity
    Answer: D

11. If you were required to place waste in the ground, which of the following would be the safest for the environment?
    A) dump
    B) sanitary landfill
    C) secured landfill
    D) sanitary dump
    Answer: C

12. Also known as the Superfund legislation is the:
    A) Resource Conservation and Recovery Act of 1976 (RCRA).
    B) Clean Air Act.
    C) Comprehensive Environmental Response, Compensation, and Liability Act (CERRLLA).
    D) Sick Building Syndrome legislation.
    Answer: C

13. Which of the following is not true about the Pollutant Standard Index (PSI)?
    A) It was created by the EPA.
    B) It relates pollutant concentrations to health effects.
    C) The higher the PSI, the better the air quality.
    D) All of the above are not true.
    Answer: C

14. Most of the acid rain in the United States is created in what part of the country?
    A) Northeast
    B) Southwest
    C) Midwest
    D) Southeast
    Answer: C

15. What is the primary cause of the depletion of the ozone layer?
    A) global warming
    B) chlorofluorocarbons
    C) acid rain
    D) sulfur coal
    Answer: B

16. Which of the following air pollutants are considered criteria pollutants in the United States?
    A) carbon monoxide and lead
    B) nitrogen dioxide and ozone
    C) particulate matter and sulfur dioxide
    D) all the above
    E) just A and B
    Answer: D

17. The most important of the greenhouse gases is:
    A) nitrous oxide.
    B) chlorofluorocarbons.
    C) carbon dioxide.
    D) methane.
    Answer: C

18. Which of the following statements about thermal inversion is not true?
    A) More likely to occur around mountainous areas.
    B) Caused when warm air is trapped by cool air.
    C) Thermal inversions can trap smog.
    D) Results from warmer air trapping cooler air.
    Answer: B

19. The first Earth Day occurred on April 22, :
    A) 1815.
    B) 1915.
    C) 1956.
    D) 1970.
    Answer: D

20. All of the following are common indoor air pollutants except:
    A) asbestos.
    B) chlorofluorocarbons.
    C) formaldehyde.
    D) radon.
    Answer: B

21. Which of the following statements about Sick Building Syndrome is <u>not true</u>?
A) The concept emantes from common law.
B) Determined by production of signs and symptoms of ill health.
C) Became known to public health officials in mid-1970s.
D) Can occur outside too.
Answer: D

22. The endless movement of water from the earth's surface, to the atmosphere, and back to the earth's surface is called:
A) aquifer movement.
B) the hydrologic cycle.
C) the desalinization movement.
D) the water cycle.
Answer: B

23. Which of the following statements about water is <u>not true</u>?
A) Most of the world's water supply has salt in it.
B) Most of the world's water supply is found in the oceans.
C) The largest store of fresh water is found in rivers.
D) Removing salt from water is an expensive process.
Answer: C

24. All of the following are examples of non-point pollution <u>except</u>:
A) runoff of chemicals from farm fields.
B) seepage of leachates from landfills.
C) the release of pollutants by a factory into a stream.
D) acid rain.
Answer: C

25. Which of the following statements about the Clean Water Act is <u>not true</u>?
A) Aimed at ensuring all rivers were swimmable and fishable.
B) It was the first comprehensive federal water quality law.
C) The only federal legislation that deals with drinking water.
D) Aimed at reducing the discharge of pollutants into the United States waters to zero.
Answer: C

26. Which stage of waste water treatment is considered a physicial/mechanical process?
A) primary
B) secondary
C) tertiary
Answer: A

27. At what stages of waste water treatment is sludge produced?
A) primary and secondary
B) primary and tertiary
C) secondary and tertiary
Answer: A

28. At what stage of waste water treatment would one likely find a comminutor?
    A) primary
    B) secondary
    C) tertiary
    Answer: A

29. It was not until 1988 that this stage of waste water treatment was required of sewage treatment plants by the Environmental Protection Agency.
    A) primary
    B) secondary
    C) tertiary
    Answer: B

30. What percent of all Americans dispose of their waste water via a septic system?
    A) 5
    B) 25
    C) 50
    D) 75
    Answer: B

31. The major components of a septic system are:
    A) absorption field and sludge pump.
    B) absorption field and septic tank.
    C) septic tank and comminutor.
    D) sludge pump and comminutor.
    Answer: B

32. Which of the following statements about noise is _not true_?
    A) Unwanted sound is referred to as noise.
    B) Sound is the by-product of the conversion of energy.
    C) Frequency is measured by decibels.
    D) Amplitude refers to sound volume, loudness, or intensity.
    Answer: C

33. The one pollution in the United States that receives the least attention is:
    A) air.
    B) water.
    C) noise.
    D) hazard wastes.
    Answer: C

True-False

Write T if the statement is true and F if the statement is false.

1. Interactions between humans and the environment are referred to as ecology.
   Answer: True

2. An example of nutritive energy is heating oil.
   Answer: False

3. An example of non-nutritive energy is food.
   Answer: False

4. The geophysical system is comprised of the Earth; its water, and its atmosphere.
   Answer: True

5. A diverse biosphere is more stable than one with fewer species.
   Answer: True

6. Whether chemicals are considered chemical hazards depends upon their toxicity.
   Answer: True

7. The Resource Conservation and Recovery Act of 1976 and its amendments provide for "cradle-to-grave" regulation of solid and hazardous wastes.
   Answer: True

8. Leachates are liquids created when water mixes with the wastes in landfills.
   Answer: True

9. Dumps and sanitary landfills are different words for the same method of waste disposal.
   Answer: False

10. Incineration reduces considerably the weight and volume of solid waste.
    Answer: True

11. One reason why Americans have been slow to recycle is the inconvenience of doing so.
    Answer: True

12. One reason why Americans have been slow to recycle is the lack of incentives to do so.
    Answer: True

13. Composting is a complicated process that can only be done by experienced environmentalists.
    Answer: False

14. The ultimate means of dealing with solid waste is to limit its creation in the first place.
    Answer: True

15. All but 10 states in the United States have "bottle bills".
    Answer: False

16. The Superfund was created primarily to cleanup abandoned hazardous waste sites.
    Answer: True

17. The lower the Pollutant Standard Index (PSI), the poorer the air quality.
    Answer: False

18. Chlorofluorocarbons naturally occur in the environment.
    Answer: False

19. Global warming is the gradual increase in temperature of the air surrounding the earth.
    Answer: False

20. The first National Clean Air Act was passed in 1815.
    Answer: False

21. Asbestos is a naturally occurring mineral fiber that was commonly used as an insulation and fireproofing material.
    Answer: True

22. Mainstream smoke is the smoke that comes off the end of a burning tobacco product.
    Answer: False

23. It has been postulated that banning smoking probably would save more lives than any other pollution control measure.
    Answer: True

24. Underground reservoirs of water are referred to as aquifers.
    Answer: True

25. Virtually all surface water is polluted and needs to be treated before it can be safely consumed.
    Answer: True

26. Less than 2% of all water treated for human consumption is used for drinking or cooking.
    Answer: True

27. Waste water is the substance that remains after water has been used or consumed by humans.
    Answer: True

28. Most treatment facilities in the United States do not have capabilities to perform tertiary treatment of waste water.
    Answer: True

29. Radon gas is the biggest contributor to terrestrial radiation.
    Answer: True

30. At the present time in the United States, there is no public waste facility capable of handling high level nuclear wastes.
    Answer: True

31. Presently, there is no alternative to burying high level nuclear wastes.
    Answer: False

32. The most effective noise policies are those developed at the local level where they address specific noise issues.
    Answer: True

Essay

Write your answer in the space provided or on a separate sheet of paper.

1. What were some of the environmental issues that were raised during the American presidential campaign of 1992?
   Answer: (1) locating and opening new landfills; (2) long term solutions for wastes; (3) protecting the spotted owl; (4) environment constraints on new factories; (5) global warming

2. Identify four factors that have contributed to an increasing number of environmental hazards.
   Answer: (1) urbanization; (2) industrialization; (3) population growth; (4) the production and use of disposable products and containers

3. What problem is represented in the 1987 Islip, New York, garbage problem?
   Answer: We are generating waste faster than we can dispose of it in an environmentally sound way.

4. What are the major differences between a dump and a sanitary landfill?
   Answer: A dump is an open pit in the ground where waste is placed. A sanitary landfill is located on a site that can geographically and geologically support it. Waste is compacted and covered with soil in a landfill.

5. Explain the major drawbacks of the incineration of municipal waste.
   Answer: (1) incinerators are expensive to build; (2) some air pollution; (3) disposal of remaining ash; (4) toxicity of remaining ash; (5) impedes recycling

6. What are the primary problems associated with acid deposition?
   Answer: (1) acidification of surface water resulting in death to certain species of water life; (2) damage to vegetation primarily in the higher elevations; (3) the erosion of monuments and buildings; (4) reduced visibility; (5) possibly respiratory problems in humans

7. Explain how ozone is both a help and harm to human health.
   Answer: At ground level ozone gas is considered a criteria pollutant, however, in the stratosphere it serves as a filter of the sun's harmful ultraviolet rays.

8. What two pieces of legislation in 1970 radically changed the course of pollution control?
   Answer: (1) The establishment of the Environmental Protection Agency and (2) Amendments to the Clean Air Act.

9. What kind of steps can be taken to reduce or eliminate indoor air pollution?
   Answer: (1) use pump dispensers instead of spray; (2) vent dryers outdoors; (3) avoid products containing formaldehyde; (4) remove loose asbestos fibers; (5) limit or prohibit indoor smoking; (6) keep furnace and air conditioners in good working order; (7) periodically test for radon

10. Identify the four steps included in the treatment of most surface water used for consumption.
    Answer: (1) coagulation and flocculation; (2) sedimentation; (3) filtration; (4) disinfection

11. What are the two primary means of improving waste water so that it is not harmful to the environment or humans?
Answer: One is by killing the pathogenic organisims that entered the waste water as part of human wastes. The second is by converting organic wastes into inorganic wastes so that they will not unduly enrich the waters receiving the treated waste water.

12. What three things insure the safety of a septic system?
Answer: It is safe if it is (1) properly located in appropriate soil, (2) carefully constructed, and (3) properly maintained.

13. Give an example of noise modification for each of the following: A. source of the noise; B. path the noise travels; C. protection for exposed parties.
Answer: (A) suppressing the origination of noise; (B) blocking the path of travel; (C) covering the ears of the exposed parties

Matching

Choose the item from Column 2 that best matches each item in Column 1.

Match the following descriptions with the appropriate component of the environmental system.

1.	traveling	human activity
2.	scrap wood and metal	residue or waste
3.	energy	life support system
4.	disease	environmental hazard
5.	recreating	human activity
6.	boredom, stress and fear	environmental hazard
7.	buildings (built environment)	life support system
8.	urine and feces	residue or waste
9.	earthquakes and floods	environmental hazard
10.	trash and garbage	residue or waste
11.	social interactions	life support system
12.	acquiring food	human activity

Match the following activities with the means of waste disposal.

13.	best solution to hazardous waste disposal	hazardous waste recycling

14. least expensive means of disposing of hazardous waste

secured landfill

15. located in impermeable rock

deep well injection

16. in Europe waste exchanges have been created to help with this

incineration of hazardous waste

17. useful for only small amounts of waste

neutralization of hazardous waste

Match the following pollutants with the appropriate category of pollutants.

18. pathogens

biological water pollutant

19. lead

toxic water pollutant

20. oil spill

miscellaneous water pollutant

21. bacteria

biological water pollutant

22. thermal pollution

miscellaneous water pollutant

23. parasites

biological water pollutant

24. pesticides

toxic water pollutant

25. overgrowth of aquatic plants

biological water pollutant

Match the following forms of radiation with its source.

26. sunlight

naturally occurring radiation-cosmic

27. nuclear medicine diagnosis

human-made radiation

28. radon gas

naturally occurring radiation-terrestrial

29. bricks and stones

naturally occurring radiation-terrestrial

30. radiation therapy

human-made radiation

31. tobacco

human-made radiation

32. smoke detectors

human-made radiation

33. dental x-rays

human-made radiation

34. nuclear power plants

human-made radiation

35. computer screens

human-made radiation

36. water from contaminated well

naturally occurring radiation-internal

Chapter 16   The Impact of Environment on Human Health

Multiple-Choice

Choose the one alternative that best completes the statement or answers the question.

1. Biological hazards can include:
    A) poison ivy or poison oak.
    B) bacteria.
    C) viruses.
    D) all the above
    E) just B and C
    Answer: D

2. Which of the following is the most likely scenario?
    A) Sanitary engineers are assisted by sanitarians.
    B) Sanitarians are assisted by sanitary engineers.
    C) Sanitary engineers and sanitarians work independently.
    D) Sanitary engineers inspect facilities and report violations of the public health code.
    Answer: A

3. Chlorination is often used as a safeguard against what type of diseases?
    A) vector-borne diseases
    B) food-borne diseases
    C) water-borne diseases
    D) air-borne diseases
    Answer: C

4. With the exceptions of botulism and chemical poisoning, how many people have to become ill for the Centers for Disease Control and Prevention to declare a food-borne outbreak?
    A) two or more
    B) five or more
    C) twenty or more
    D) fifty or more
    Answer: A

5. Which of the following can lead to food-borne disease?
    A) improper holding temperature for foods
    B) inadequate cooking
    C) consumption of shell fish from polluted waters
    D) all the above
    E) just A and B
    Answer: D

6. Standing water provides an ideal habitat for which vector?
   A) fleas
   B) mosquitoes
   C) ticks
   D) lice
   E) both B and D
   Answer: B

7. Rodents are often hosts for:
   A) fleas.
   B) mosquitoes.
   C) ticks.
   D) none of the above
   Answer: A

8. If a farmer applied a herbicide to kill weeds in a cornfield, the weeds would be referred to as:
   A) target weeds.
   B) nontarget pest.
   C) nontarget organism.
   D) target pest.
   Answer: D

9. The two groups at highest risk for pesticide poisoning are:
   A) young adults and senior citizens.
   B) young children and young adults.
   C) young children and workers who apply pesticides.
   D) children and adolescents who cannot read directions.
   Answer: C

10. Poisonings occur when the pesticides are:
    A) consumed orally.
    B) inhaled.
    C) in contact with the skin.
    D) all the above
    E) just A and B
    Answer: D

11. A persistent (long lasting) pesticide can be described as a:
    A) warm pesticide.
    B) hard pesticide.
    C) cold pesticide.
    D) soft pesticide.
    Answer: B

12. The process of breathing in environmental tobacco smoke is referred to as:
    A) second hand smoke.
    B) sidestream smoke.
    C) passive smoking.
    D) mainstream smoking.
    Answer: C

13. Which group of individuals is at highest risk for lead poisoning?
    A) youngsters
    B) adolescents
    C) young adults
    D) adults
    E) senior citizens
    Answer: A

14. Which of the following is not true about skin cancer?
    A) Appears more often on exposed body parts.
    B) Is the most common form of cancer.
    C) Appears more in dark skin people than light skin people.
    D) Has the potential to harm more people living close to the equator than those not living near
       the equator.
    Answer: C

15. The most dangerous skin cancer is:
    A) basal cell carcenomas.
    B) squamous cell carcenomas.
    C) malignant cell carcenomas.
    Answer: C

16. The highest sun protective factor endorsed by the Food and Drug Administration is:
    A) 2.
    B) 15.
    C) 30.
    D) 50.
    Answer: C

17. Which of the following statements about radon is false?
    A) It is a colorless, tasteless, odorless gas.
    B) It is formed from the decay of uranium.
    C) Humans consume it by inhaling it.
    D) It is the number one cause of lung cancer in the United States.
    E) It can enter a home through cracks in the foundation, walls and floors.
    Answer: D

18. The greatest growth in a given population is represented by which phase of the population
    s-curve?
    A) lag phase
    B) exponential phase
    C) equilibrium phase
    D) learning phase
    Answer: B

19. Which of the following community health problems are caused either in part or whole by population growth?
    A) smog and acid rain
    B) crime and depletion of the ozone layer
    C) global warming and bulging landfills
    D) all the above
    E) just A and C
    Answer: D

20. In the United States, the voluntary agency that has taken on the role to help communities recover from a natural disaster is:
    A) American Cancer Society.
    B) American Red Cross.
    C) United Way.
    D) Community Chest.
    Answer: B

True-False

Write T if the statement is true and F if the statement is false.

1. Sanitarians are public health workers who inspect facilities and report breakdowns or violations of the public health code.
   Answer: True

2. Delicatessens, cafeterias or restaurants are reported nearly twice as often as homes as places where food-borne disease resulted from consuming contaminated food.
   Answer: True

3. The number one contributing factor of outbreaks of food-borne diseases is poor personal hygiene of preparers.
   Answer: False

4. Vectors are usually insects.
   Answer: True

5. Diseases that are transmitted from humans to animals are referred to as zoonoses.
   Answer: False

6. From a biological standpoint there is no such thing as a pest.
   Answer: True

7. The two most commonly used pesticides are insecticides and rodentcides.
   Answer: False

8. The majority of the children poisoned by pesticides consume them orally.
   Answer: True

9. There is no such thing as a perfect pesticide.
   Answer: True

10. There is a cause-effect relationship between environmental tobacco smoke and ill health.
   Answer: False

11. Environmental tobacco smoke is now considered a Group A carcinogen, just like asbestos.
   Answer: True

12. Humans are exposed to lead primarily by ingestion and inhalation.
   Answer: True

13. Occupational exposure to lead is the major source of lead intake for adults.
   Answer: True

14. People can be exposed to lead if they consume water from lead pipes or pipes connected with lead solder.
   Answer: True

15. It is possible to have well water contaminated with lead.
   Answer: True

16. The lower the sun protective factor (SPF) number on sunscreens the greater the amount of protection.
   Answer: False

17. There is a fairly inexpensive (around $29) way to check your home for radon.
   Answer: True

18. Zero population growth would be characterized by equal birth and death rates.
   Answer: True

19. More than 75% of the world's population is found in developing countries.
   Answer: True

20. An earthquake is an example of a disaster agent.
   Answer: True

21. The primary needs of people after a natural disaster usually include adequate food, water, shelter, health care, and clothing.
   Answer: True

22. The key to recovery from any natural disaster lies in the ability of the federal government to provide aid.
   Answer: False

Essay

Write your answer in the space provided or on a separate sheet of paper.

1. Why is it so difficult to effectively study the impact of some environmental factors on human health?
   Answer: It is so difficult to control all the associated variables during the research process.

2. Why is rodent control an important community health service?
   Answer: Because rodents are often hosts for disease carrying vectors.

3. If a person were to use a herbicide on a flower garden, what would be considered the target and nontarget organisms?
   Answer: target -weeds; nontarget -flowers

4. How would you describe the perfect pesticide?
   Answer: (1) It would be inexpensive, (2) it would affect only the target organism, (3) it would have a short half-life, and (4) it would break down into harmless materials.

5. What concepts should be included in worksite no smoking policies?
   Answer: (1) No smoking in the workplace and disincentive for those who do, (2) provide information about health promtion and the adverse effects of smoking, (3) offer smoking cessation classes to all workers, (4) provide incentives to encourage smokers to stop. Also, make sure to include both management and labor in the policy making process.

6. Identfy three major ways to abate lead poisoning and give an example of each.
   Answer: (1) Education -provide people, especially parents, with information about the dangers of ingesting lead. (2) Regulation -many communities are now covered by laws that regulate the use of products with lead in them -gasoline for example. (3) Prudent behavior -people need to avoid behavior that would increase their chances of lead consumption -avoid the consumption of water with lead in it.

7. What individuals are at greatest risk for skin cancer?
   Answer: Those who: (1) have excessive exposure to UV radiation, (2) have fair complexions, and (3) are occupationally exposed to coal tar, pitch, creosote, and arsenic compounds or radium.

8. Explain the ABCD rule for the warning signs of melanoma.
   Answer: A is for asymmetry B is for border irregularity C is for color D is for diameter greater than 6 millimeters

9. Draw and label the population s-curve.
   Answer: Draw the s-curve; label the bottom the lag phase, the middle the exponential phase, and the top is the stable equilibrium phase.

10. What is meant by the statement "A stable population will occur either through 1) human action to conscientiously limit population growth, or 2) actions taken by nature to limit population growth via survival of the fittest?"
    Answer: There are limited amounts of resources on Earth and humankind can either use them wisely or let nature determine who will and who will not survive.

Matching

Choose the item from Column 2 that best matches each item in Column 1.

Match the following diseases with their method of transmission.

1.	Lyme disease	vector-borne disease
2.	typhus	vector-borne disease
3.	typhoid fever	water-borne disease
4.	botulism	food-borne disease
5.	polio	water-borne disease
6.	St. Louis encephalitis	vector-borne disease
7.	Rocky Mountain Spotted fever	vector-borne disease
8.	cholera	water-borne disease

Chapter 17   Injuries as a Community Health Problem

Multiple-Choice

Choose the one alternative that best completes the statement or answers the question.

1. Unintentional injuries include those resulting from:
   A) car crashes and falls.
   B) assaults and suicides.
   C) drownings and fires.
   D) just A and B
   E) just A and C
   Answer: E

2. The term accident has fallen into disfavor and disuse with many public health officials and now has been replaced with the term:
   A) unintentional injury.
   B) intentional injury.
   C) injury abuse.
   D) Injury mishap.
   Answer: A

3. Which of the following would be considered an unsafe condition?
   A) Driving an automobile while being impaired by alcohol.
   B) icy streets
   C) Operating a power saw without eye protection.
   D) None of the above are unsafe conditions.
   Answer: B

4. Injury is the _____ leading cause of death in the United States.
   A) 1st
   B) 2nd
   C) 3rd
   D) 4th
   Answer: D

5. Approximately what percent of Americans are involved in some type of motor vehicle crash each year?
   A) 40
   B) 30
   C) 20
   D) 10
   Answer: D

6. Unintentional injuries is the leading cause of death for which age group?
   A) birth to 44 years of age
   B) birth to 65 years of age
   C) 32 to 54 years of age
   D) 16 to 50 years of age
   Answer: A

7. Which of the following groups are at high risk for death by unintentional firearm injury?
   A) infants and children
   B) children and teenagers
   C) teenagers and adults
   D) adults and older adults
   Answer: B

8. The death rates resulting from unintentional injury is highest in which race?
   A) Asian Americans
   B) Black Americans
   C) Native Americans
   D) White Americans
   Answer: C

9. The single most important risk factor for unintentional injuries is:
   A) age.
   B) gender.
   C) alcohol.
   D) race.
   E) place.
   Answer: C

10. Safety belt laws are an example of what type of approach to unintentional injury prevention?
    A) education
    B) regulation
    C) automatic protection
    D) litigation
    Answer: B

11. Interpersonal violence disproportionately affects which of the following?
    A) Those who are frustrated and hopeless.
    B) Those who are jobless and live in poverty.
    C) Those with low self-esteem.
    D) all the above
    E) just A and B
    Answer: D

12. The rates of suicide in young people (15 to 24 years of age) have _ since 1950.
    A) decreased
    B) stayed the same
    C) doubled
    D) tripled
    Answer: D

13. _____ is the failure of a parent or guardian to care for or otherwise provide the necessary subsistence for a child.
    A) Child abuse
    B) Child neglect
    C) Child emotional abuse
    D) Child physical abuse
    Answer: B

14. Two primary reasons behind the increased numbers of gang related deaths are:
    A) violence on television and lack of discipline in schools.
    B) drug trafficking and abuse, and the availability of firearms.
    C) firearms and reduction in the police force.
    D) crowded jails and prisons and increased number of gangs.
    Answer: B

15. It was recommended that a comprehensive approach to violence prevention should address which of the following areas:
    A) firearms violence.
    B) alcohol and other drugs.
    C) childhood experiences and mental disorders that put people at high risk.
    D) all the above
    E) just A and B
    Answer: D

True-False

Write T if the statement is true and F if the statement is false.

1. Hazards do not cause unintentional injuries.
   Answer: True

2. Injury is the leading cause of death in the United States.
   Answer: False

3. Injury is the leading cause of lost productivity in the United States.
   Answer: True

4. More people die from unintentional injuries associated with motor vehicle crashes than any other type of injury.
   Answer: True

5. About twice as many male deaths can be attributed to unintentional injury than female deaths.
   Answer: True

6. While more injuries occur on the road, more deaths occur at home.
   Answer: False

7. The primary thesis behind public health legislation to prevent unintentional injuries is "for the good of the total public."
   Answer: True

8. The homicide rate in the United States is significantly lower than in other industrialized nations.
   Answer: False

9. More violent acts are committed by males than females.
   Answer: True

10. Black males are more likely to die on the streets of a major American city today than an American soldier was to die in Vietnam.
Answer: True

11. Violence in America has steadily declined since 1985.
Answer: False

12. The most common child abuse is sexual abuse.
Answer: False

13. The most common category of child neglect is educational neglect.
Answer: True

14. The best approach against gang violence is a multi-faceted effort.
Answer: True

15. A key to reducing violence in a community seems to be to empower communities to develop their own violence prevention programs.
Answer: True

Essay

Write your answer in the space provided or on a separate sheet of paper.

1. Identify the four characteristics of unintentional injury.
   Answer: (1) Occurs following an unplanned event, (2) is usually preceded by an unsafe act or condition (hazard), (3) is often accompanied by economic loss or injury, and (4) interrupts the efficient completion of a task.

2. How did each of the following contribute to early injury prevention and control: Hugh De Haven, John E. Gordon, and William Haddon, Jr.?
   Answer: Hugh De Haven -studied victims of falls in an effort to design ways to reduce the force of impact on a body. John E. Gordon -proposed in 1949 that the tools of epidemiology be used to analyze injuries. William Haddon, Jr. -the founding father of modern injury control. He was the foremost expert on highway safety in the 1960s.

3. Using the model of unintentional injuries, label the triangle below using the example of injury resulting from a motor vehicle crash on an icy road.
   Answer: Triangle -top is environment (icy road), bottom right corner is host (automobile passenger), bottom left corner is agent (energy).

4. Based upon the model for unintentional injuries, there are four types of actions that can be taken to prevent or reduce the number and seriousness of unintentional injuries and deaths. Name the four and give an example of each.
   Answer: Examples are not provided because there are many possibilities. (1) Prevention of the accumulation of the injury producing agent, energy, (2) prevention of the inappropriate release of excess energy or modify its release in some way, (3) placement of a barrier between the host and agent, and (4) separation of the host from the potentially dangerous sources of energy.

5. Give an example for each of the four broad strategies for the prevention of unintentional injuries; education, regulation, automatic protection, and litigation.
   Answer: (1) Education -fire drills, lessons on bicycle safety and other safety lessons (2) Regulation -speed limits, safety belt laws, motorcycle helmet laws, laws about fences around swimming pools (3) Automatic protection -child proof safety caps, air bags and automatic safety belts (4) Litigation -any court case resulting in safer behavior

6. Why is it stated that interpersonal violence has a tremendous economic cost on the community?
   Answer: So many resources are needed to deal with it such as the police, the legal system, the penal system, emergency health care services, health care services, social wokers and many more.

7. What are the three components of the model for abuse?
   Answer: abuser, abused and crisis

8. Identify the major approaches to preventing intentional injuries.
   Answer: (1) Education, (2) providing better opportunities for employment and recreation, (3) regulation and enforcement, and (4) improving social services.

9. Why is it so difficult to pass legislation to control health behavior?
   Answer: (1) personal freedom, (2) jeopardize or otherwise interfere with legal activities that provide livelihood for some

Matching

Choose the item from Column 2 that best matches each item in Column 1.

Match the time periods with the appropriate unintentional injuries.

1. from May to August	most drownings occur
2. from January to April	fewer motor vehicle deaths occur
3. from October to March	most deaths resulting from fire
4. at night	more motor vehicle deaths occur
5. during the day	fewer motor vehicle deaths occur
6. on the weekends	more motor vehicle deaths occur

Match the following activities with the appropriate type of abuse or neglect.

7. hitting another person	physical abuse
8. rape	sexual abuse
9. burning a child with a cigarette	physical abuse
10. shaking another person	physical abuse

11. obscene phone calls   sexual abuse

12. failure to provide warmth   emotional abuse

13. indecent exposure   sexual abuse

14. teasing of another person   verbal abuse

15. failure to provide attention   emotional abuse

16. fondling a child   sexual abuse

17. failure to provide food   child neglect

18. failure to keep a child clean   child neglect

Chapter 18   Safety and Health in the Workplace

Multiple-Choice

Choose the one alternative that best completes the statement or answers the question.

1. Occupational diseases and injuries result from:
    A) spending too much time at work.
    B) exposure to something in the work environment.
    C) illegal use of substances in the work place.
    D) over exposure to some substance.
    Answer: B

2. Each year in the United States:
    A) more people die from occupational injuries than occupationally related diseases.
    B) more people die from occupationally related diseases than occupational injuries.
    C) deaths from occupational injuries is about equal to the number of deaths from occupationally related diseases.
    Answer: B

3. What do Bhopal, India, Three Mile Island in the United States, and Chernobyl, Russia, all have in common?
    A) All had great loss of life do to an industrial disaster.
    B) All were sites of industrial disasters.
    C) All were impacted by the meltdown of nuclear reactors.
    D) All were sites of industrial disasters with United States companies involved.
    Answer: B

4. Which state was first to pass laws concerning hazards in the workplace in 1835?
    A) Virgina
    B) Ohio
    C) Indiana
    D) Massachusetts
    Answer: D

5. Alice Hamilton (1869-1970), a true pioneer of occupational health, led crusades to reduce occupational poisonings from:
    A) coal dust.
    B) heavy metals such as lead and mercury.
    C) textile dust.
    D) machine oil in the cotton mills.
    Answer: B

6. Which of the following was (were) created by the Occupational Safety and Health Act of 1970?
    A) Occupational Safety and Health Administration (OSHA)
    B) National Institute of Occupational Safety and Health (NIOSH)
    C) Department of Labor
    D) just A and B
    E) just A and C
    Answer: D

7. Which of the following is __not__ true about the Occupational Safety and Health Act of 1970?
    A) It established the Occupation Safety and Health Administration.
    B) It allows employees the right to request an OSHA inspection.
    C) It made OSHA responsible for recommending occupational and safety standards.
    D) It established the National Institute of Occupational Safety and Health.
    E) It requires employees to follow specific safety and health standards.
    Answer: C

8. The leading cause of occupational injury deaths is:
    A) electricity.
    B) falls.
    C) motor vehicle crashes.
    D) machinery.
    Answer: C

9. The number one job related nonfatal injury is:
    A) head injuries.
    B) hand injuries.
    C) back injuries.
    D) eye injuries.
    Answer: C

10. Which of the following __is true__ about occupational injuries?
    A) Female workers are injured more than male workers.
    B) Older workers are injured more than young workers.
    C) White Americans have higher occupational death rates than workers of color.
    D) Asian Americans have the lowest occupational death rates.
    Answer: D

11. The highest job related death rates are found among:
    A) timber cutters/loggers and pilots.
    B) construction workers.
    C) farmers.
    D) race car drivers and pilots.
    Answer: A

12. Which of the following __is not__ a means of reducing injuries on the job?
    A) Modifying the job to make it safer.
    B) Changing the work environment to be less hazardous.
    C) Taking migrant workers out of the fields and placing them in factories.
    D) Improving the selection, training and education of the worker.
    Answer: C

13. The safety worker that is most concerned about radiation safety in the workplace is:
    A) safety engineers.
    B) certified safety professionals.
    C) health physicist.
    D) industrial hygienists.
    Answer: C

14. _____ are concerned with environmental factors that might cause disease.
    A) Safety engineers
    B) Certified safety professionals
    C) Health physicists
    D) Industrial hygienists
    Answer: D

15. What factor (factors) drive workplace health promotion programs?
    A) To promote the health of the employee.
    B) The personal concern employers have for employees.
    C) The impact of the health of the employee and employee families on the corporation, and community.
    D) all the above
    E) just B and C
    Answer: D

16. _____ are those portions of the workplace health and safety program aimed at reducing the number and seriousness of unintentional injuries on the job.
    A) Health promotion programs
    B) Safety programs
    C) Disease prevention programs
    D) Employee assistance programs
    Answer: B

True-False

Write T if the statement is true and F if the statement is false.

1. Next to home, Americans spend the next largest portion of their time at work.
   Answer: True

2. The occupation fatality rate in the United States is higher than those in Sweden, Japan or Germany.
   Answer: True

3. Progress in occupational health legislation moved very quickly in the first half of the twentieth Century.
   Answer: False

4. The purpose of the Occupational and Health Safety Act of 1970 was to provide a working environment free of hazards that are causing or likely to cause death or serious physical harm.
   Answer: True

5. Under the Occupational Safety and Health Act of 1970, an employee has the right to request an OSHA inspection.
   Answer: True

6. The job related injury that accounts for the greatest cost from worker's compensation claims is hand injuries.
Answer: False

7. Studies show that those living in countries where income is lower have significantly lower occupational death rates than those living in higher income countries.
Answer: False

8. There is a seasonality to work related deaths.
Answer: True

9. All tractors manufactured since 1985 are fitted with safety belts and roll over protective structures.
Answer: True

10. The most effective means of reducing injuries on the job is to make machinery safer.
Answer: False

11. Acute trauma refers to single exposure injuries, while cumulative trauma is the result of several exposures.
Answer: True

12. The greatest number of cases of skin disorders occurs in agriculture.
Answer: False

13. Proving that an agent at the workplace is the cause of a reproductive problem is very difficult.
Answer: True

14. There is little formal training in occupational medicine in most medical schools.
Answer: True

15. Over 80% of United States' worksites with 50 or more employees offer some form of a health promotion program.
Answer: True

Essay

Write your answer in the space provided or on a separate sheet of paper.

1. Why do the estimates on occupational injuries and injury deaths vary considerably?
   Answer: Several different organizations/agencies (National Center for Health Statistics, National Safety Council, Bureau of Labor Statistics, and the National Institute for Occupational Safety and Health) provide statistics on the topic.

2. Why are migrant farm workers at such high risk for health problems?
   Answer: (1) Exposure to chemical and biological hazards, (2) poor water quality, (3) long exposure to the sun, (4) poor access to health care, and (5) many children working.

3. Using the epidemiological model (agent-host-environment), identify several different means of controlling occupational diseases.

Answer: (1) Identification and evaluation of agents, (2) standard setting for handling and exposure to causative agents, (3) elimination or substitution of causative factors, (4) engineering controls to provide for a safer work area, (5) environmental monitoring, (6) medical screening, (7) personal protective devices, (8) health promotion, (9) disease surveillance, (10) therapeutic medical care and rehabilitation, and (11) compliance activities.

Matching

Choose the item from Column 2 that best matches each item in Column 1.

Use the letter A through G to put in chronological order (oldest to most recent) the events of the history of occupational safety and health.

1. George Agricola's treatise on mining   A

2. Alice Hamilton   F

3. Industrial Revolution   B

4. Child Labor Law   D

5. Occupational Safety and Health Act   G

6. inspection of workplaces for sanitation and cleanliness   C

7. Workers' Compensation Laws   E

Match the following health problems with the appropriate classification.

8. skin cancer   dermatogical condition

9. silicosis   lung disease

10. leading cause of occupational disease fatalities   occupational cancers

11. coal worker's pneumoconiosis   lung disease

12. back injury   musculoskeletal

13. asbestosis   lung disease

14. tendinitis   musculoskeletal

15. impacts largest organ of   dermatogical
     the body   condition

16. result from inhalation of   lung diseases
     toxic substance

17. leading cause of disability   musculoskeletal
     in the work force

Match the following lung problems with the correct descriptor.

18. brown lung   byssinosis   asbestosis

19. black lung   coal worker's   asbestosis
                                  pneumoconiosis

20. dust on lungs   silicosis   asbestosis

TRANSPARENCY MASTERS

TRANSPARENCY MASTERS

to accompany

McKenzie/Pinger
INTRODUCTION TO COMMUNITY HEALTH

Transparency Master No.	Transparency Master Title	Text Figure
TR-1	Important rates in Epidemiology	Table 3.4
TR-2	Cases of Specified Notifiable Diseases	Table 3.5
TR-3	Secular display: Incidence of poliomyelitis by year, United States 1951-1991	3.5
TR-4	Seasonal (cyclical) epidemiologic graph	3.6
TR-5	Point source epidemic curve: Cases of gastroneteritis following ingestion of a common food source	3.7
TR-6	Propogated epidemic curve: Cases of chicken pox during April-June	3.8
TR-7	Causative Agents for Disease and Injury	Table 4.1
TR-8	School Health Services	6.5
TR-9	Recommended schedule of vaccinations for all children, 1993	Table 8.9
TR-10	Selected international comparisons	Box 9.6
TR-11	General adaptation syndrome	11.3
TR-12	Consequences of drug use	Table 12.1
TR-13	Percentage of high school seniors who have used drugs - class of 1992	Table 12.2
TR-14	Types of health insurance coverage	Table 14.2
TR-15	Inventory of recommended available services appropriate to a long-term care support system	14.7
TR-16	HMO model types	14.8
TR-17	Categories of services used in the prioritization process	Box 14.4
TR-18	The environmental system	15.1
TR-19	Reusable versus throwaway goods	Table 15.1
TR-20	Diagram of a secured landfill	15.10

TR-1 Important rates in Epidemiology

Important Rates in Epidemiology

Rate	Definition	Examples (U.S. 1992)
Crude birth rate	$\dfrac{\text{Number of live births}}{\text{Estimated midyear population}} \times 1{,}000$	16.0/1,000
Crude death rate	$\dfrac{\text{Number of deaths (all causes)}}{\text{Estimated midyear population}} \times 1{,}000$	8.5/1,000
Age-specific death rate	$\dfrac{\text{Number of deaths, 35–44}}{\text{Estimated midyear population, 35–44}} \times 1{,}000$	2.3/1,000
Infant mortality rate	$\dfrac{\text{Number of deaths under 1 year of age}}{\text{Number of live births}} \times 1{,}000$	8.5/1,000
Neonatal mortality rate	$\dfrac{\text{Number of deaths under 28 days of age}}{\text{Number of live births}} \times 1{,}000$	5.4/1,000
Cause-specific death rate	$\dfrac{\text{Number of deaths (diabetes mellitus)}}{\text{Estimated midyear population}} \times 100{,}000$	17.2/100,000

TR-2 Cases of Specified Notifiable Diseases

Summary—Cases of Specified Notifiable Diseases, United States, Cumulative, Week Ending December 26, 1992 (52nd week)[6]

	Cum. 1992		Cum. 1992
AIDS	42,978	Measles:	
Anthrax	1	Imported	130
		Indigenous	2,068
Botulism: foodborne	19	Plague	12
Infant	59		
Other	4	Poliomyelitis, paralytic	—
Brucellosis	87	Psittacosis	86
Cholera	102	Rabies, human	—
Congenital rubella syndrome	9	Syphilis, primary and secondary	32,637
Diphtheria	4	Syphilis (congenital) age <1 yr	1,639
Encephalitis, post-infectious	108	Tetanus	39
Gonorrhea	471,488	Toxic shock syndrome	218
Haemophilus influenzae-flu		Trichinosis	39
(invasive disease)	1,222	Tuberculosis	22,592
Hansen disease	148	Tularemia	153
Leptospirosis	46	Typhoid fever	376
Lyme disease	7,777	Typhus fever, tick-borne (RMSF)	489

TR-3 Secular display: Incidence of poliomyelitis by year, United States 1951-1991

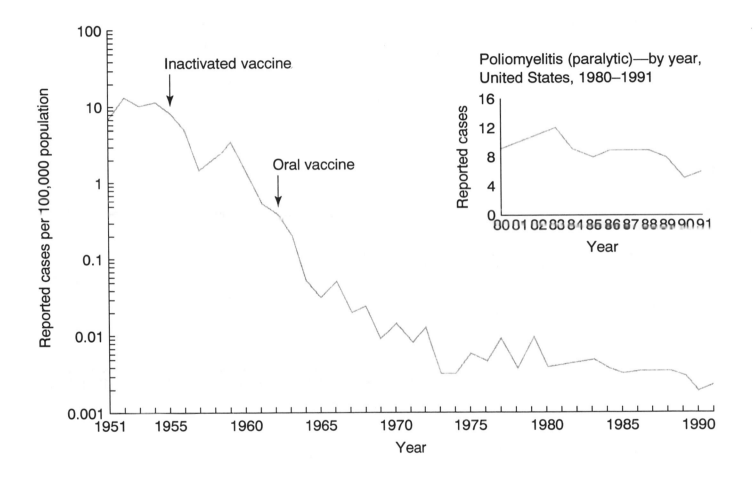

TR-4 Seasonal (cyclical)epidemiologic graph

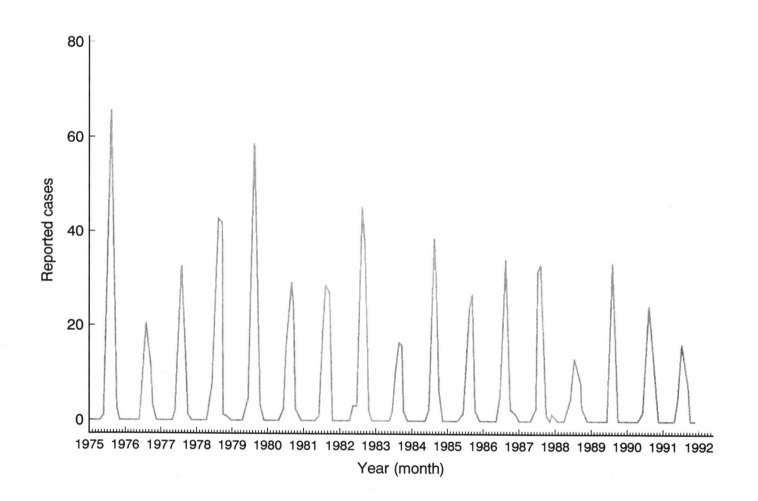

TR-5 Point source epidemic curve: Cases of gastroneteritis following ingestion of a common food source

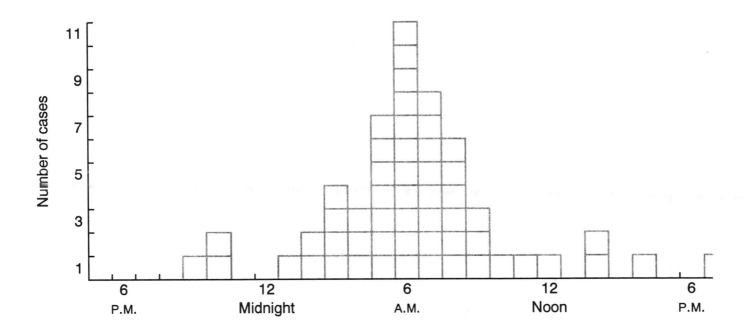

TR-6 Propogated epidemic curve: Cases of chicken pox during April-June

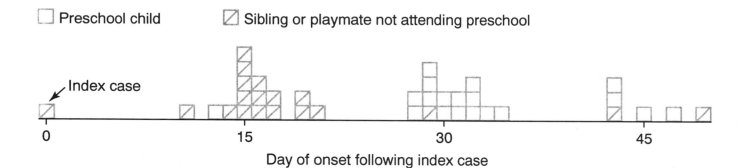

Causative Agents
for Diseases and Injuries

Biological Agents	Chemical Agents	Physical Agents
Viruses	Pesticides	Heat
Rickettsiae	Food additives	Light
Bacteria	Pharmacologics	Radiation
Fungi	Industrial chemicals	Noise
Protozoa	Air pollutants	Vibration
Metazoa	Cigarette smoke	Speeding objects

TR-8 School Health Services

Comprehensive Health
Reproductive health care
Acute diagnosis and treatment
Acute and chronic illness management
Laboratory testing
STD testing and treatment
Family planning information and referral
Prenatal and pediatric care
Dental screenings and services

Expanded Health
Health promotion/disease prevention
Mental health counseling
Drug and alcohol counseling/prevention education
Health, family life, and sex education
Case management (ensuring continuum of care)
Care of special-needs children

Basic Health
EPSDT screenings
Immunizations
Hearing/vision screenings
Scoliosis screening
Emergency care
Sports physicals
Health counseling
Nutrition screenings

Recommended Schedule of Vaccinations for All Children, 1993

Age	DTP	DTaP	OPV	MMR	Hib Option 1[1]	Hib Option 2[1]	HBV Option 1	HBV Option 2
Birth	...	...	...	...	...	...	X	...
2 months	X	...	X	...	X	X	X[2]	X[2]
4 months	X	...	X	...	X	X	...	X[2]
6 months	X	...	...	...	X	...	...	...
12 months	...	...	...	...	...	X	...	...
15 months	X[3]	X[3]	X[3]	X[4]	X	...	...	...
6–18 months	...	...	...	...	...	...	X[2]	X[2]
4–6 years (before school)	X	X	...	X[5]	...	...	...	...

[1]Vaccine is given in either a 4-dose schedule in option 1 or a 3-dose schedule in option 2, depending the type of vaccine used.

[2]Hepatitis B vaccine can be given simultaneously with DTP, OPV, MMR, and Hib at the same visit.

[3]Many experts recommend these vaccines at 18 months.

[4]In some areas, this dose of MMR may be given at 12 months.

[5]American Academy of Pediatrics recommends that this dose be given at entry to middle school or junior high school.

Note: DTP = Diphtheria, tetanus, and pertussis vaccine; DTaP = Diphtheria, tetanus, and acellular pertussis vaccine; OPV = Live oral polio vaccine; MMR = Measles, mumps, and rubella vaccine; Hib = Haemophilus b conjugate vaccine; HBV = Hepatitis B vaccine.

From: Robinson, C. A., S. J. Sepe, and K. F. Y. Lin (1993). "The President's Child Immunization Initiative—A Summary of the Problem and the Response." *Public Health Reports* 108(4): 420.

BOX 9.6
Selected International Comparisons

Indicators		Canada	France	Germany*	Japan	United Kingdom	United States
Percentage of low-birth-weight babies	1990	6	5	6	6	7	7
Infant mortality rate (per 1,000 live births)	1990	6.8	7.4	7	4.6	7.9	9.1
Teen birth rate (per 1,000 teens) (1988)	Selected years	23.1 (1988)	9.5 (1988)	10.3 (1988)	3.5 (1989)	31.8 (1989)	54.8
Percentage of appropriate age group enrolled in secondary education	1988–1989	93	83	85	96	79	88
Percentage of all deaths that are violent deaths, ages 15–24 (1986)	Selected years	76.2 (1986)	70 (1986)	68.7 (1987)	66.5 (1987)	62.3 (1987)	77.8
Percentage of children in poverty (1987)	Selected years	9.6 (1987)	4.6 (1984)	2.8 (1984)	—	7.4 (1986)	20.4
Percentage of all households that are married couples with children (1988)	Selected years	32.3 (1986)	30.2 (1988)	21.8 (1988)	39.2 (1985)	28 (1987)	27
Percentage of all households that are single-parent households (1988)	Selected years	5.6 (1986)	3.7 (1988)	3.4 (1988)	2.5 (1985)	4 (1987)	8

*Germany for low birth-weight and infant mortality statistics; former West Germany for all others.

From: No author (1993). *Kids Count Data Book*. Greenwich, Conn.: The Annie E. Casey Foundation, and Washington, D.C.: Center for the Study of Social Policy.

TR-11 General adaptation syndrome

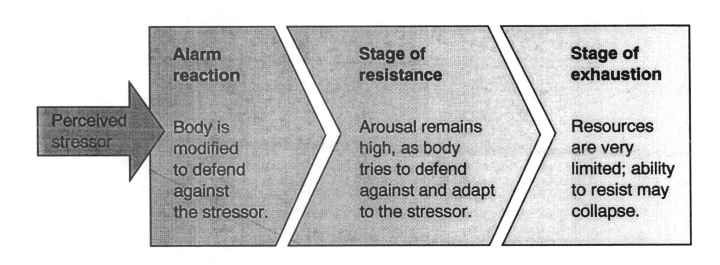

Perceived stressor

Alarm reaction

Body is modified to defend against the stressor.

Stage of resistance

Arousal remains high, as body tries to defend against and adapt to the stressor.

Stage of exhaustion

Resources are very limited; ability to resist may collapse.

TR-12 Consequences of drug use

Consequences of Drug Use

Personal Consequences	Community Consequences
Absenteeism from school or work	Loss of productivity and revenue
Underachievement at school or work	Lower average SAT scores
Scholastic failure/interruption of education	Loss of economic opportunity
Loss of employment	Increase in public welfare load
Marital instability/family problems	Increase in number of broken homes
Risk of infectious diseases	Epidemics of sexually transmitted diseases
Risk of chronic or degenerative diseases	Unnecessary burden on health care system
Increased risk of accidents	Unnecessary deaths and economic losses
Financial problems	Defaults on mortgages, loans/bankruptcies
Criminal activity	Increased cost of insurance and security
Arrest and incarceration	Increased cost for police/courts/prisons
Risk of adulterated drugs	Increased burden on medical care system
Adverse drug reactions or "bad trips"	Greater need for emergency medical services
Drug-induced psychoses	Unnecessary drain on mental health services
Drug overdose	Unnecessary demand for medical services
Injury to fetus or newborn baby	Unnecessary use of expensive neonatal care
Loss of self-esteem	Increase in mental illness, underachievement
Suicide	Damaged and destroyed families
Death	

TR-13 Percentage of high school seniors who have used drugs – class of 1992

Percentage of High School Seniors Who Have Used Drugs— Class of 1992

	Ever Used	Past Month	Daily Use
Alcohol	87.5%	51.3%	3.4%
Cigarettes	61.8	27.8	17.2
Marijuana	32.6	11.9	1.9
Stimulants	13.9	2.8	0.2
Inhalants	16.6	2.3	0.1
Cocaine	6.1	1.3	0.1
Tranquilizers	6.0	1.0	*
Hallucinogens	9.2	2.1	0.1
Sedatives	6.1	1.2	0.1
Crack	2.6	0.6	0.1
PCP	2.4	0.6	0.1
Heroin	1.2	0.3	*

*Less than 0.05%

From: Johnston, L. D., P. M. O'Malley, and J. G. Bachman (1993). National Survey Results on Drug Use from the "Monitoring the Future Study," 1975–1992. Vol. I: "Secondary School Students" (NIH pub. no. 93-3597). Washington, D.C.: U.S. Government Printing Office.

TR-14 Types of health insurance coverage

Types of Health Insurance Coverage

dental—Dental procedures.

disability—Income when insured is unable to work because of a health problem.

hospitalization—Inpatient hospital expenses including room, patient care, supplies, and medications.

major medical—Large medical expenses usually not covered by regular medical or dental coverage.

optical—Nonsurgical procedures to improve vision.

regular medical—Nonsurgical service provided by health care providers. Often has set amounts (fixed indemnity for certain procedures).

surgical—Surgeons' fees (for inpatient or outpatient surgery).

TR-15 Inventory of recommended available services appropriate to a long-term care support system

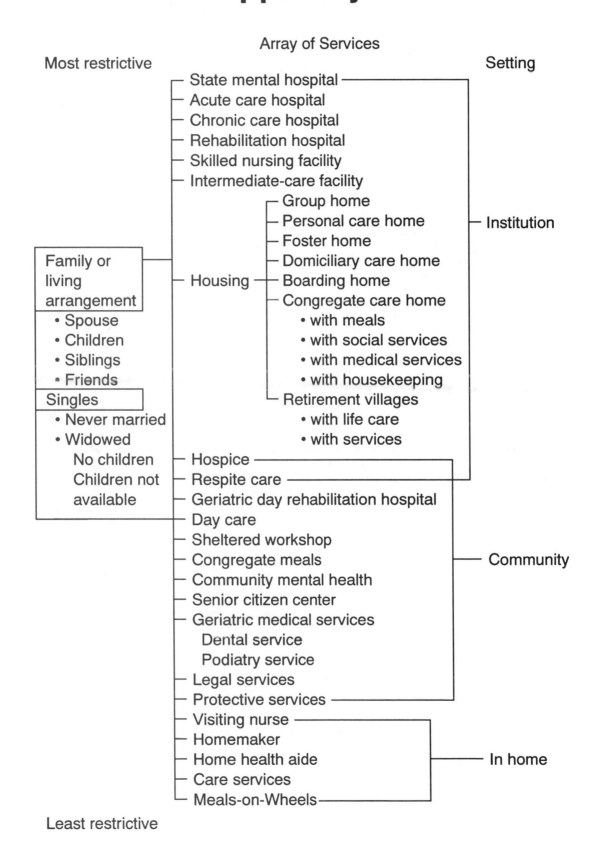

Array of Services

Most restrictive

Setting

State mental hospital
Acute care hospital
Chronic care hospital
Rehabilitation hospital
Skilled nursing facility
Intermediate-care facility

Group home
Personal care home
Foster home
Domiciliary care home
Housing — Boarding home
Congregate care home
• with meals
• with social services
• with medical services
• with housekeeping
Retirement villages
• with life care
• with services

Institution

Family or living arrangement
• Spouse
• Children
• Siblings
• Friends

Singles
• Never married
• Widowed
  No children
  Children not available

Hospice
Respite care
Geriatric day rehabilitation hospital
Day care
Sheltered workshop
Congregate meals
Community mental health
Senior citizen center
Geriatric medical services
  Dental service
  Podiatry service
Legal services
Protective services

Community

Visiting nurse
Homemaker
Home health aide
Care services
Meals-on-Wheels

In home

Least restrictive

TR-16 HMO model types

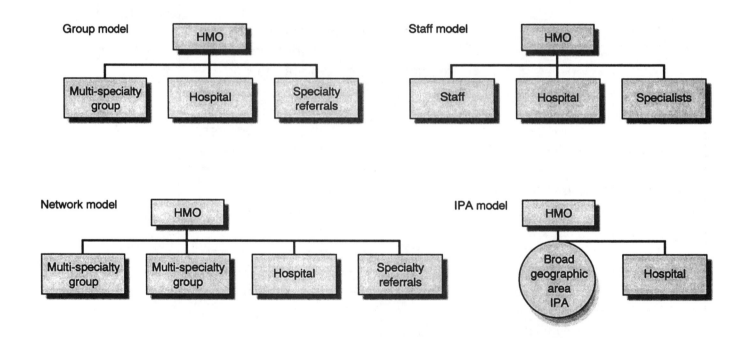

Group model

HMO

Multi-specialty group

Hospital

Specialty referrals

Staff model

HMO

Staff

Hospital

Specialists

Network model

HMO

Multi-specialty group

Multi-specialty group

Hospital

Specialty referrals

IPA model

HMO

Broad geographic area IPA

Hospital

TR-17 Categories of services used in the prioritization process

BOX 14.4
Categories of Services Used in the Prioritization Process and Examples of Condition-Treatment (CT) Pairs

Category	Description
"Essential" services	
1. Acute fatal	Treatment prevents death with full recovery. Example: appendectomy for appendicitis.
2. Maternity care	Maternity and most newborn care. Example: obstetrical care for pregnancy.
3. Acute fatal	Treatment prevents death without full recovery. Example: Medical therapy for acute bacterial meningitis.
4. Preventive care for children	Example: Immunizations.
5. Chronic fatal	Treatment improves life span and quality of life. Example: Medical therapy for asthma.
6. Reproductive services	Excludes maternity/infertility services. Example: Contraceptive management.
7. Comfort care	Palliative therapy for conditions in which death is imminent. Example: Hospice care.
8. Preventive dental care	Adults and children. Example: Cleaning and fluoride applications.
9. Proven effective preventive care for adults	Example: Mammograms.
"Very important" services	
10. Acute nonfatal	Treatment causes return to previous health state. Example: Medical therapy for vaginitis.
11. Chronic nonfatal	One-time treatment improves quality of life. Example: Hip replacement.
12. Acute nonfatal	Treatment without return to previous health state. Example: Arthroscopic repair of internal knee derangement.
13. Chronic nonfatal	Repetitive treatment improves quality of life. Example: Medical therapy for chronic sinusitis.
Services that are "valuable to certain individuals"	
14. Acute nonfatal	Treatment expedites recovery of self-limiting conditions. Example: Medical therapy for diaper rash.
15. Infertility services	Example: In-vitro fertilization.
16. Less effective preventive care for adults	Example: Screening of nonpregnant adults for diabetes.
17. Fatal or nonfatal	Treatment causes minimal or no improvement in quality of life. Example: Medical therapy for viral warts.

Source: Oregon waiver application, Aug. 1991.

From: Congress of the United States, Office of Technology Assessment (May 1992). *Summary: Evaluation of the Oregon Medicaid Proposal* (pub. no. OTA-H-532). Washington, D.C.: U.S. Government Printing Office, p. 6.

TR-18 The environmental system

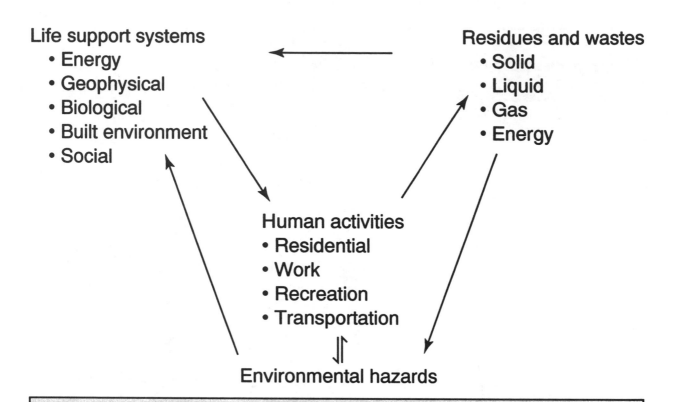

Life support systems
- Energy
- Geophysical
- Biological
- Built environment
- Social

Residues and wastes
- Solid
- Liquid
- Gas
- Energy

Human activities
- Residential
- Work
- Recreation
- Transportation

Environmental hazards

Site and location
- Earthquakes
- Floods
- Wind Storms
- Drought

Biological
- Animal
- Insect
- Microbiological
- Vegetation

Chemical
- Poisons and toxins
- Allergens
- Irritants

Physical
- Vibration
- Radiation
- Forces and abrasion
- Humidity

Psychological
- Stress
- Boredom
- Anxiety
- Discomfort
- Depression

Sociological
- Overcrowding
- Isolation
- Anomie

Reusable Versus Throwaway Consumer Goods

Reusable Goods	*Throwaway Goods*
Milk bottles	Cardboard cartons and plastic jugs
Returnable soft drink bottles	Aluminum cans and plastic bottles
Cloth diapers	Disposable diapers
Garbage cans	Trash bags
Lunch boxes	Paper bags
Cloth napkins	Paper napkins
Refillable pens	Disposable pens
Handkerchiefs	Facial tissues
Cloth towels or rags	Paper towels
Ceramic or plastic dishes	Paper plates

TR-20 Diagram of a secured landfill

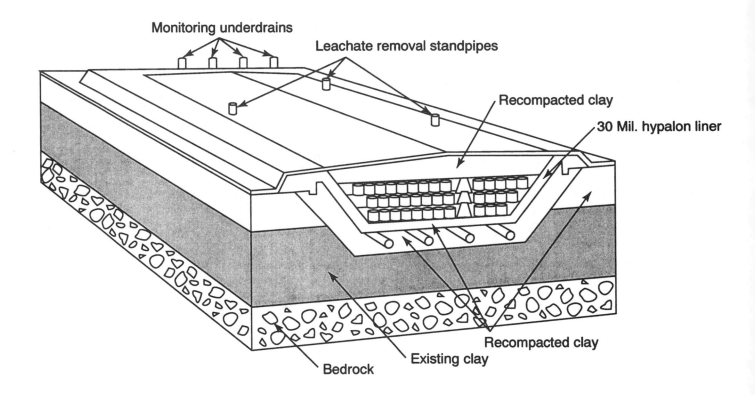

Monitoring underdrains

Leachate removal standpipes

Recompacted clay

30 Mil. hypalon liner

Recompacted clay

Existing clay

Bedrock

TR-21 Criteria pollutants

Criteria Pollutants

Pollutants (Designation)	Form(s)	Major Sources (in order of percentage of contribution)
Carbon monoxide (CO)	Gas	Transportation, industrial processes, other, solid waste, stationary fuel combustion.
Lead (Pb)	Metal or aerosol	Transportation, industrial processes, stationary fuel combustion, solid waste.
Nitrogen dioxide (NO_2)	Gas	Stationary fuel combustion, transportation, industrial processes, solid waste, other.
Ozone (O_3)	Gas	Transportation, industrial processes, solid waste, other, stationary fuel combustion.
Particulate matter (total suspended particles—TSP)	Solid or liquid	Industrial processes, stationary fuel combustion, transportation, solid waste, other.
Sulfur dioxide (SO_2)	Gas	Stationary fuel combustion, industrial processes, transportation, other.

TR-22 Sunscreen guide

Sunscreen Guide

Skin Type	Pigmentation	Sunburn/Tanning History	Sun Protection Factor (SPF)
1.	Very fair skin; freckling; blond, red, or brown hair	Always burns easily; never tans	15–30
2.	Fair skin; blond, red, or brown hair	Always burns easily; tans minimally	15–20
3.	Brown hair and eyes, darker skin (light brown)	Burns moderately; tans gradually and uniformly	8–15
4.	Light brown skin; dark hair and eyes (moderate brown)	Burns minimally; always tans well	8–15
5.	Brown skin; dark hair and eyes	Rarely burns, tans profusely (dark brown)	Recommend same as Skin type 4
6.	Brown-black skin; dark hair and eyes	Never burns, deeply pigmented (black)	Recommend same as Skin Type 4

Note: As deterioration of the ozone layer continues, it may be necessary to use an even more protective sunscreen.

From: Payne, W. A., and D. B. Hahn (1992). *Understanding Your Health,* 3rd ed. St. Louis: Mosby Yearbook, p. 329.

TR-23 A theoretical population curve—S-curve

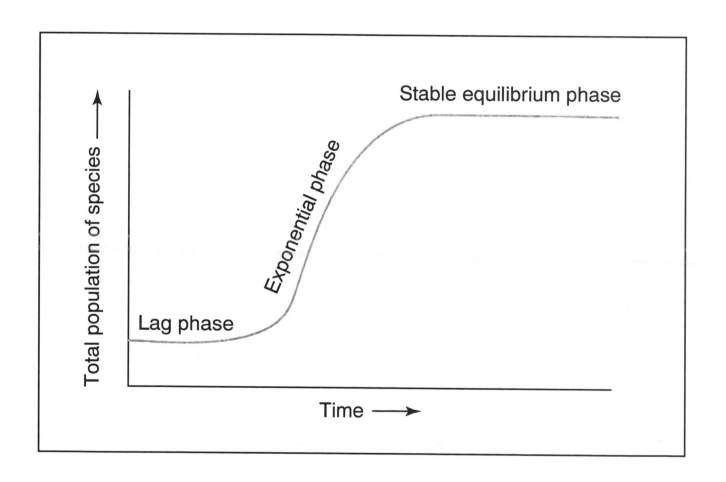

TR-24 A population curve—J-curve

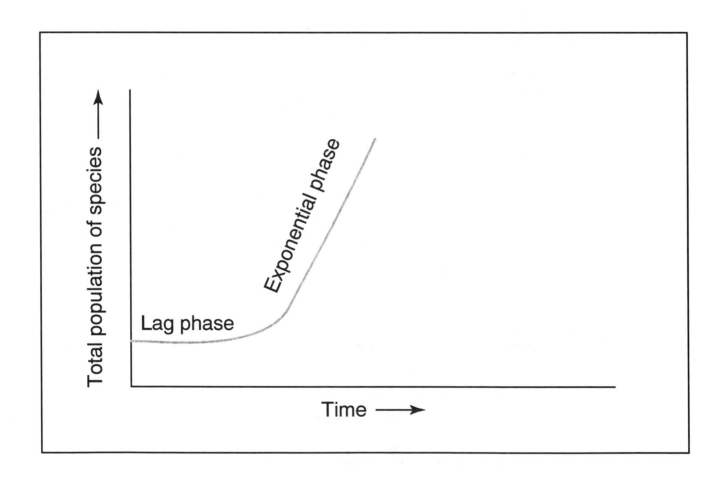

TR-25 Attenuation of the effect of a public health education program

Total target population $n = 100$

Those exposed to educational messages $n = 66$

Those who comprehend messages $n = 44$

Those who change behaviors $n = 29$

Those whose new behaviors persist over time $n = 19$

Those who apply new behavior to prevent injury at moment of risk $n = 13$

Those for whom injury is prevented or reduced as a result of applying behavior at moment of risk $n = ?$